LIFE, LIBERTY
AND THE PURSUIT OF
SEXUAL HEALTH

WESTON M. EDWARDS, PH.D.

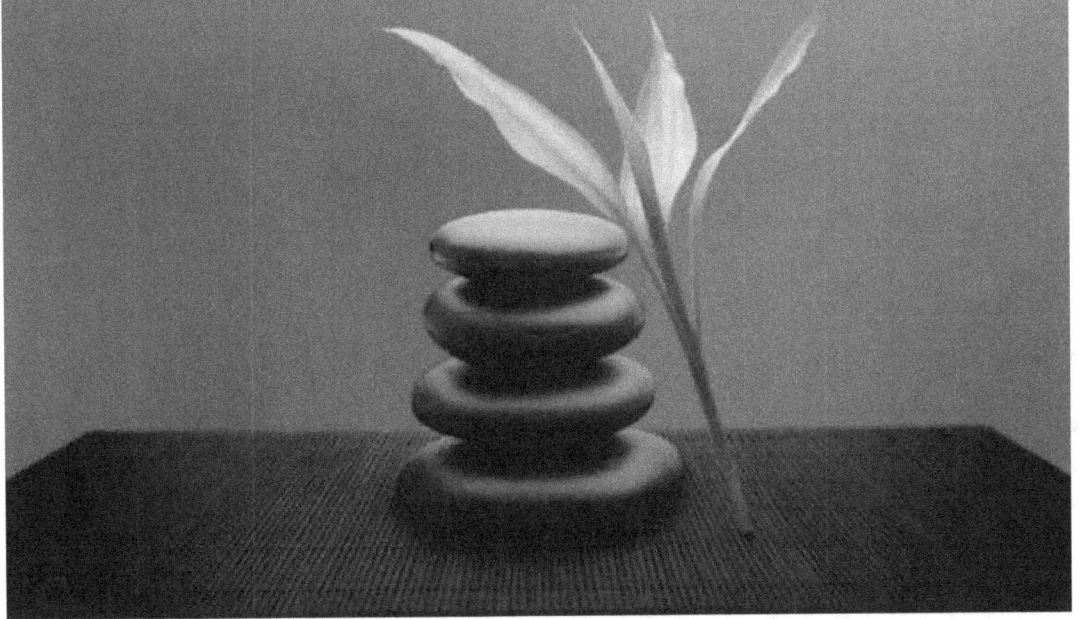

Copyright Page

Life, Liberty and the Pursuit of Sexual Health

Contact Information

Weston Edwards, PhD

Email: Weston@westonmedwards.com

For additional copies of this workbook, please visit or email

www.livingalifeilovebooks.com

www.sexualhealthinstitute.org

LifeILove@sexualhealthinstitute.org

Disclaimer. This information provides accurate and authoritative information regarding sexuality; the information is for education purposes only. The publisher and author are not engaged in providing professional services. You should seek the services of a trained professional if you need expert assistance or therapy services.

Table of Contents

LIFE, LIBERTY AND THE PURSUIT OF SEXUAL HEALTH 1
INTRODUCTION 1
THE POWER OF STORY 2
THE POWER AND EXPERIENCE OF SEXUAL HEALTH 3
TOWARD YOUR PERSONAL DEFINITION OF SEXUAL HEALTH 4
THE TEN COMPONENTS OF THE SEXUAL HEALTH MODEL 5
FIVE CORE TASKS 7
WHY DOES A PERSON STOP AT A STOP SIGN? THE ROLE OF INQUIRY. 8
STRUCTURE OF THE ASSIGNMENTS 8
DISCERNMENT 9
A PROGRAM OF INTEGRITY 10
THE POWER OF PARALLEL PROCESS 12
THE PAIN OF SEXUALITY 13
THE "REVERSE-GOLDEN-RULE." 14
HOW (NOT) TO USE THIS BOOK 15
LIFE COACHING AND SEXUAL HEALTH 15
FINDING A SEX THERAPIST 16
THE IMPORTANCE AND LIMITS OF CONFIDENTIALITY AND RISK OF DISCLOSURE 17

CHAPTER 1: TALKING ABOUT SEX 18
HOW COMFORTABLE ARE YOU? 19
REVIEWING YOUR SEX HISTORY 21
SEXUAL BEHAVIOR TIMELINE 28

CHAPTER 2: CULTURE, VALUES AND STEREOTYPES 33
POWER OF THOUGHT 33
CULTURE AND STEREOTYPES 36
   Feelings of Shame and Guilt 44
SEXUAL IDENTITY AND SEXUAL ORIENTATION 47

CHAPTER 3: PHYSICAL COMPONENTS OF SEXUAL HEALTH 55
WHAT IS SEXUAL FUNCTIONING 55
GENERAL TYPES OF SEXUAL DYSFUNCTION ISSUES 57
SEXUAL FUNCTIONING AND DEVELOPMENT OF SEXUAL SKILLS 59
TYPES OF SEXUAL INTIMACIES 61
SAFER-SEX ISSUES 64

CHAPTER 4: BARRIERS TO SEXUAL HEALTH 68
   Sexual Compulsivity: what is compulsive? 68
   Sexual Avoidance 69
   Chemical Dependency 69
   Eating Disorders 71
MENTAL HEALTH FACTORS 72
   ADHD 73

Depression 74
Bipolar Disorder/Manic Depression 75
Anxiety 77
TREATMENT FOR MOOD DISORDERS 78
TYPES AND IMPACT OF ABUSE 81
USE OF THE INTERNET AND OTHER TECHNOLOGY 90
BEHAVIORAL ANALYSIS 91

CHAPTER 5: INTERNAL FACTORS OF SEXUAL HEALTH **93**
BODY IMAGE 93
DEVELOPING A HEALTHY BODY IMAGE 95
WHAT WOULD YOUR GENITALS SAY? 97
MASTURBATION 98
FANTASY 101
SEXUALLY EXPLICIT MATERIAL 105

CHAPTER 6: POSITIVE SEXUALITY **108**
POSITIVE SEXUALITY 108
WHY HAVE SEX? 109
ASSERTIVE COMMUNICATION 110
BOUNDARIES 113
SEXUAL BEHAVIOR AND EXPRESSION 116
HISTORICAL DEFINITIONS OF HEALTH SEXUAL EXPRESSION 117

CHAPTER 7: INTIMACY AND RELATIONSHIPS **123**
DESIRE FOR INTIMACY 123
TYPES OF INTIMACY 123
TOUCH/PHYSICAL INTIMACY 129
BARRIERS TO INTIMACY 130
DATING AND SEXUAL HEALTH 132
THE LANGUAGE OF RELATIONSHIPS 134
RELATIONSHIP SATISFACTION 135
HEALING FROM PAST RELATIONSHIPS 136
STEPS IN BUILDING THE SEXUAL RELATIONSHIP 137
TYPE OF RELATIONSHIPS 144
FEELINGS OF GRIEF 148
FINDING A RELATIONSHIP THERAPIST 151

CHAPTER 8: SPIRITUALITY, VALUES AND SEXUAL HEALTH **152**
BARRIERS TO SPIRITUALITY 152
POWER OF STORY 153

A NEW BEGINNING: CONTINUING THE CONVERSATION **160**
THE NEXT STEP 160
SEXUALHEALTHINSTITUTE.BLOGSPOT.COM 160
ADDITIONAL RESOURCES 161
END NOTES 164

Life, Liberty and the Pursuit of Sexual Health

Introduction

Everything is connected to sexuality. A broad statement, yet I believe that all of our living is built on sex and sexuality. Simply look around the environment and it is possible to see connections to sexuality. Most advertising is built on sexuality: "If I buy this thing, I will get the right partner, perfect job, or woo the person of my dream." The funniest jokes are often based on sexual innuendo. Two of the biggest social issues of the day are related to sexuality: same-sex relationships and abortion. Many of our fears about the future involve the question of whether or not we will find someone to love. Some of the biggest uncertainties in life are about trusting our partner and fearing that our partner might leave us. Our biggest existential pains are connected to relationship failures. The biggest scandals in the mainstream media are often sex focused.

These examples highlight how important sexuality is in our life. But almost nowhere do we have any discussion about sexuality that fosters growth and understanding. There are not a lot of resources available to foster sexual health. In our culture, much of the discussion on sexual health is "unspoken," i.e., it is not discussed openly. Or, when spoken, the discussion is fear-based and shame-based. Almost all of the larger conversations around sexuality are this way. The term to describe this typical approach is "sex-negative."

This book takes a different approach. What would it look like to expand the discussion on sexuality and "hear" all the messages we hear about sexuality? What would it look like if we sat down and discussed our sexual health issues with the important people in our life? What would it look like if each of us identified what is healthy in our life and actually took the responsibility to assertively get our needs met? What would a sex-positive approach to sexuality look like?

The purpose of this workbook is to help individuals discover and address specific topics to help them move toward improved sexual health. The topics reflect what I think the research suggests are the most important topics. The information is simply the tip of the iceberg. I encourage you to seek out and find additional support and information. The rest of the introduction discusses how to use the contents of the book. My hope is that your find the journey toward sexual wellness challenging and even enjoyable.

The Power of Story

When we think about who we are, we essentially come up with a story. When you string enough of the stories together, you develop a sense of self. Some of our stories have a profound role in shaping our identity; other stories have a minimal impact. Sometimes there is a story we want to deny, avoid or otherwise minimize. Sometimes we simply forget our stories. In a few cases, we've never thought about a particular story line. When prompted, however, thinking about the story can lead to profound change.

I encourage you to think of all of the stories you have about yourself and others. One place to look for your stories is the phrase that comes after "because." "I do that because…. I'm that way because… This is important because…" These are the stories that shape your life.

As you will find, some of the stories may be helpful or unhelpful. Some stories may suggest topics to review with your support network or therapist. A few of the stories may be a source of profound joy or emotional pain. As you understand the stories, there is no right or wrong story. What is important is that this is your story. All of our beliefs about sexuality are based on these stories.

Believe it or not, it is possible to change the story. This is a process of growth and development. Taking a new perspective on a story can lead to new insights. Gaining additional information changes the content of the story. Feedback from peers can facilitate a reframing of the story. This process of change requires us to know and understand the stories in our life. The movement toward sexual health is the process of discovering our stories of sexuality. The workbook is designed to help you rewrite and update your stories of sexuality.

The Power and Experience of Sexual Health

A mentor (someone whom I greatly respect) and I have a running discussion concerning the need to *learn* about sexual health versus the need to *experience* sexual health. While we might argue the nuances, I think we agree that both are important. Much of this workbook is about providing basic education regarding sexual health. I am impressed with HOW MUCH individuals want to understand sexual health. Here are some thoughts on how to move forward in your experience of sexual health.

- Give yourself permission to be a sexual being. Sexuality is a normal, vital, and positive aspect of your life. Too many people suffer pain when they think about sexuality.

- Ask, "Says who?" One of the earliest questions a child learns is "why?" Plenty of stories are available where eventually an exhausted parent says, "Because, I said so and eat your carrots!" The question applies in the realm of sexuality. We have been told the "truth" about sexuality with the explanation, "Because I said so." Challenge most, if not all, of the messages you have heard about sexuality. This doesn't mean you have to discard your beliefs. Instead, understand both the letter and spirit of the messages.

- Sexual Health is a journey. Today's thoughts are for today. What you like today is for today. What you want is for today. Too often we lose sight of today, and "catastrophize" every sexual experience.

- Reach out for support. Using your support network best facilitates the process. The network can include friends, family or professionals such as your therapist, spiritual guide, or other providers.

- Balance is important in the journey. Too often we look ONLY for perfection, and if perfection is not possible, the experience is BAD, SINFUL, and UNHEALTHY. Sexual health recognizes many variables. For example, I place good/bad sexual experiences on a different continuum than the continuum of healthy/unhealthy. You can have a sexual encounter that feels good but is unhealthy (think meth/sex), and a bad experience that is healthy (think too tired to function, but emotional intimacy).

- Experiment. When you watch a child in a playground, they meander through all of the play areas. They might stop at the swings, or the merry go around. Next, they may check out the slide, and perhaps build something in the sand. When they like something, the child stays in the area. If a bully or something is unpleasant, the child moves on. So, too, is it important to experiment in the realm of sexuality. Check out what you like or don't like. Enjoy the positive experiences, and let go of the unpleasant experiences.

Enjoy your journey in sexual health. My hope is that you have great experiences along the way. Sometimes the only way we know what is sweet is because we understand what is sour.

Toward Your Personal Definition of Sexual Health

Through your work in the assignments, you will uncover a personal definition of sexual health that reflects your life, values and circumstances. The focus of the assignments is to help your discern YOUR truth regarding sexuality. My experience suggests that if you are a client, you are much more successful with sexual wellness when it reflects YOUR truth. What do you really want in your life? Much of what we believe is based on what we are told we SHOULD want. Listen to the language in statements by others; the frequency of "You SHOULD…." is amazing. All of our marketing is based on "You SHOULD." Much of our sexuality discussion is based on "you should," or often, "You shouldn't."

I invite you to increase your awareness in all the ways you are told, "I should," or "shouldn't" or, even when you say, "I should" or "I shouldn't." In reality, anything is possible. Sexual health requires that you choose and declare, "I choose to live my life this way; I choose to engage in or not engage in these behaviors." There is a significant pressure toward conformity in sexuality. It is your responsibility to assertively confront this pressure. What you choose is truly your choice.

What is sexual health? There are a number of formal definitions, but in the end, it is simply authenticity. It is neither good, nor bad, it is simply authentic. And it is YOUR authenticity, not what you think others think should be authentic to you. Yes, that reads awkwardly, but the key is to focus on your authenticity. People often worry so much about what family, friends, partners, and others think is important that they lose their voice.

Authenticity is more than simply doing what you want when it comes to sexuality; it is engaging in behaviors that express the core of who you are. The key for you is your core, your heart of hearts. From that core, sexual health is authentic.

The Ten Components of the Sexual Health Model

To help you move toward sexual health, the topics in this workbook are based on a model of sexual health, which is briefly summarized here.[1] You will be addressing these topics throughout the workbook.

Talking About Sex

This is a cornerstone of the Sexual Health Model that includes talking about one's own sexual values, preferences, attractions, history and behaviors.

Culture, Values and Stereotypes

In order to understand a sense of sexual self, individuals must examine the impact their particular cultural heritage has on their sexual identities, attitudes and behaviors.

Sexual Anatomy and Functioning

One needs a basic understanding, knowledge and acceptance of sexual anatomy, sexual response and sexual functioning. Sexual health includes freedom from sexual dysfunction and other sexual problems.

Sexual Health Care and Safer Sex

There are many components to this, including knowing one's body, administering regular self-exams and responding to physical changes with appropriate medical intervention. Examining one's safer sex behaviors is critical.

Challenges and Barriers to Sexual Health

Some of the major challenges include sexual abuse, substance abuse and compulsive sexual behavior. Others include sex work, harassment and discrimination.

Body Image

This requires challenging the notion of one narrow standard of beauty and encouraging self-acceptance. In order to achieve sexual health one needs to develop a realistic and positive body image.

Masturbation, Fantasy and Sexually Explicit Material

Masturbation and fantasy can each be healthy expressions of sexuality. It is important for individuals to clarify their values on these subjects. Too often, shame is linked with masturbation and fantasy because of the historical myths associated with sin, illness and immaturity.

Positive Sexuality

All human beings need to explore their sexuality in order to develop and nurture who they are within a positive and self-affirming environment. Positive sexuality includes appropriate experimentation, sensuality, sexual boundaries and sexual competence developed through the ability to give and receive sexual pleasure.

Intimacy and Relationships

Taking many forms, intimacy is a universal need that people receive through relationships. Sexual health requires knowing what intimacy needs are important for the individual, and finding appropriate ways to meet these needs. Sexual health includes learning the necessary skills to develop a variety of intimate relationships.

Spirituality, Values and Sexual Health

When there is sexual health, there is consistency between one's ethical, spiritual and moral beliefs and one's sexual behaviors. Spirituality may include identification with a formal religion, but it doesn't have to.

Five Core Tasks

Through the work in the workbook, I have my agenda. I want you to address the following five core tasks.

1) **Identify and clarify your sexual needs.** Sexual needs are defined as a desire, appetite, biological necessity, impulses, interest, and/or libido with respect to sex. How much sex do you want, what are your levels of interest, etc.

2) **Identify and clarify your sexual values.** Sexual values are defined as moral evaluations, judgments, and/or standards about what is appropriate, acceptable, desirable, and innate sexual behavior. You are the ultimate judge of what is healthy in your life.

3) **What do you like?** I want you to be able to describe what you like about sexuality and sexual expression. You will be able to identify the behaviors you like to engage in, as well as your motivations relating to or based on sexual attraction, sexual arousal, sexual gratification, or reproduction (e.g., fantasy, holding hands, kissing, masturbation, sexual intercourse).

4) **Whom do you like?** I want you to be able to identify whom you like in all realms of intimacy. What are the physical, emotional, intellectual, interpersonal, economic, spiritual, or other attributes of a sexual partner?

5) **How do you let others know?** This involves developing skills in letting others know your responses to the previous four tasks. Communication can occur via assertive communication, or learning other ways to assertively express what you want in your life.

The above tasks are the core tasks of the workbook. Everything revolves around them and eventually returns to them. All of the assignments, topics, and activities are founded on these tasks.

Why does a person stop at a stop sign? The role of inquiry.

One of my favorite exercises is to ask, "Why does a person stop at a stop sign?" After a moment of confusion often based on the thought "what is the purpose of that stupid question," the person will usually respond with a nice answer that is sometimes punctuated with an attitude (and for drama, a nice roll of the eyes) of "that is so obvious." My enjoyment is to follow-up with "Why ELSE might a person stop at a stop sign?" And the exercise continues until the person exhausts all of his/her responses (usually at about 2-3 responses). Then I ask them to think of a funny reason, a silly reason, a stupid reason, an absurd reason, etc. In one group setting, the group eventually identified 41 reasons why a person might stop at the stop sign – and my point was made: 1) Until you think outside the box, your options are limited. 2) There is more than one reason that a person stops at a stop sign. 3) Ultimately, it doesn't matter why you stop, simply that you stop. 4) You choose the reason that reflects why you stop.

So often in the realm of sexuality, we assume we know the answer to the question. We've been so taught, told, indoctrinated, forced, or otherwise encouraged to "know" the right answer, that we haven't even thought about our response to the question, "what is sexually healthy for me." The movement toward sexual health is a process of discovery and thinking outside the box. Your purpose in this process is to ask, "Why do I think this?" What else may be an answer, response, thought, issue, concern associated with the topic? This process is about unfolding, uncovering, and discovery. In the end, you are a sexual being who chooses how to be sexually healthy.

Structure of the Assignments

The tone of this workbook is conversational in nature, as if you and I were sitting together discussing the topics. Within each topic are clear-cut tasks designed to help increase your sexual health. Space is provided to answer the questions. You may find that some assignments do not apply to you, so please adapt the process to your particular needs. I encourage you to review each assignment asking yourself, "How does this topic apply to me?" Then, if the topic fits, you will need to follow-up as necessary.

As a note of caution, you may experience various levels of personal distress while working on the assignments, such as embarrassment, shame or guilt. This is typical in any personal growth process. I recommend that you have a support system to help smooth the progress of your work. This support can include a therapist, sponsor or self-help group.

Discernment

Discernment is the exercise of discovering, and revealing the truth within you. Discernment is a process. Although the first response to a question might "seem" like the "correct" response, discovering your personal truth occasionally requires additional time. Often we edit or limit our thoughts, beliefs and desires. Discovering your deeper self requires you to challenge the thoughts, beliefs and values you assume to be true. Self-identity is about integrating results from many trials and errors, experimentation, successes and failures.

Discernment is also about responsibility. It requires you to step-up and say, "This is important. This is what I believe." Too often, people avoid this responsibility for any number of fears including fear of judgment, or disapproval. Paradoxically, when you step-up and take responsibility for your journey, freedom is possible, resulting in a feeling of empowerment to say, "Yes, this is me!"

I provide three examples of the role of discernment. Staying in or leaving a relationship is a process of discernment. It is uncovering, revealing and discovering the health of the relationship. It requires an honest evaluation of your contribution to the state of the relationship, and assessment whether you are capable or willing to help build, repair or develop the relationship. It requires assessing whether the relationship can be transformed or declaring it should end.

My second example is asking what it means to live as a lesbian, gay, bisexual or transgender (LGBT) individual. There are many cultural factors (religious, family, community) that affect this process. In the end, the individual is charged with discovering what it means for him/her to live as an LGBT individual. I've seen it all. From an individual who knew at age 12 they were LGBT and appeared to have little difficulty in the process of living as an LGBT individual to a 70-year-old man coming out and choosing to stay with his wife of many decades.

My third example is linking discernment to sexual behavior. Ultimately it is up to you to determine what behaviors are sexually healthy. In other words, what behaviors help you grow as an individual, foster respect in your life and the life of your partner and the health of your community? It is a process to discover the behaviors that reflect and protect the values you use to shape your life.

A Program of Integrity

Many people want their clinician to be in charge. I cannot tell you how many times I've heard, "Tell me what to do," "Is this OK?" or "What should be my bottom-line behavior?" As a clinician, I provide feedback and suggestions, but impose very few behavioral restrictions. When I do, the restrictions are usually around legal, ethical or health consequences. I might say, "Engaging in anonymous sex with individuals isn't consistent with what you say you want," or, "Using the work computer to look at porn may get you fired."

This workbook will not tell you what to do, or have you follow a predetermined pattern of required rules. To fall into the trap of telling you right from wrong sets up the therapist as the external control. In motivational psychology, a long-term consequence of external control is a decrease in compliance with the external limits. Slowly, resentment builds as the individual "fights" with those external limits. Eventually a total break may occur where the other person's resistance causes a rupture in the therapeutic relationship.

Rather, my approach emphasizes integrity. The approach implies an internal source of control. Research in motivational psychology has repeatedly demonstrated that individuals will create profound changes and new possibilities when internally motivated; they will, for example, run marathons because they want to make a difference in the world. Think for a moment about someone who inspires you; this person's source of motivation is probably internally focused.

My approach helps you create integrity in your life. The goal is to help identify behaviors, attitudes and goals that lead to wholeness, completeness and unity. This approach, however, requires more work than simply following a list of rules. It also requires some trial and error that results in a reassessment of how you want to live your life. Following this approach, you can create an internal moral code of sexual health. You'll be happier, more effective and ultimately "whole." In the end, the approach requires from you a transformation rather than a compliance with a set of rules. In this transformation, unlimited possibilities are achievable, including living a life you love.

A number of important characteristics are identifiable by a person living in integrity.

Honesty

You say what you mean and you mean what you say. When someone asks, "How are you today?" you do not respond with a bland response. You respond with integrity by saying, "It's a good day" or "It's a bad day." In the realm of sexuality, it is saying what you mean, and meaning what you say.

Completeness

Your responses are complete. You share everything as appropriate versus disclosing parts of the response. When something happens, you are thorough about what occurred. You actively volunteer all information, versus playing a cat and mouse game about not disclosing information.

Assertiveness

Integrity requires you to speak your opinion and beliefs. If your friend, partner, support network, group or even your therapist wants you to do something, but you don't want to, the key is to be assertive in your communication. When I see a person struggling with a goal, I ask, "Are you sure it is YOUR goal?" Are you ready to put in the work toward reaching the goal? For example, do you really want to lose the five pounds, or are you simply bowing to the pressures of culture saying you "SHOULD" be skinnier when in fact you really don't want to do what is necessary regarding diet and exercise. Or like the husband who wouldn't stop viewing pornography. That wasn't his goal; it was his wife's.

Balance

Integrity reflects balance, and it is generally something we know intuitively. If something feels out of whack, you generally know it. When you ride a bicycle, for example, you know when you are in balance. The same is true for the realm of integrity. You know intuitively when you are in balance.

Endurance

Living with integrity will be tough; it will require energy to keep going when you feel like giving up. When in conflict, a desire to run away is normal but endurance requires us to stay in the conversation even when anxious or fearful.

The Power of Parallel Process

Picture a railroad track. When you look at one rail, it's pretty easy to guess where the second rail goes. Even if you see the railroad track disappear into the horizon, you have a pretty good guess that if you find one of the tracks; you'll find the other track nearby. This is what we mean by the concept of parallel process.

Often, individuals early in the discovery process express fear and anxiety about the way things will end up. I use parallel process to help people grasp where they are going when they start the therapy process. It provides a tool to shape the direction of therapy.

As an example, someone in chemical dependency recovery understands the process of recovery. A client will experience shame and guilt when they first realize they have a chemical use problem. The shame and guilt leads to isolation and increased problems. Once they start telling the stories of their chemical use, the shame and fear starts to ease and the recovery process gains momentum. Connections are made to individuals with similar struggles. Eventually recovery and a sense of hope are born allowing for a sense of being fully alive to develop.

In the same way, dealing with sexual health follows a parallel process. At the beginning, feelings of shame and guilt lead to isolation. Healing occurs through sharing your story and reaching out for support. Hope is born in the relationships and connections with others. Following the process of recovery in chemical dependency can give us a direction of recovery in sexual health.

As you start the recovery process, certain topics may be easy to talk about; and others will become easy as you continue the process. You can take your experience on the early topics and apply them to the later topics. Such is the power of parallel process.

The Pain of Sexuality

Shortly after writing my first workbook, *Living a Life I Love,* I started this edition. The workbook was inspired by someone telling me, "I don't have a problem, but I want to learn more." "I struggle with some of the topics, but I'm not compulsive/addictive/avoidant, simply unhappy in the realm of sexuality." While people used *Living a Life I Love*, it wasn't really the best fit. Thus started this workbook. (This workbook was a bit delayed as my colleagues and I finished *Cybersex Unplugged* addressing problematic online behaviors.)

I am keenly reminded of the pain many people experience in the realm of sexuality. This pain is from a variety of sources including the typical sources of abuse, shame, and guilt. But, the sources of pain can include social, familial, cultural or religious messages. A major concern is when the external messages become internalized and the individual replicates and reinforces the painful messages in a tighter and tighter circle within himself or herself. Once this pattern begins, the pain takes on a life of its own, leading to feelings of hopelessness, desperation and profound isolation. For me, this is perhaps the saddest part of the pain.

I cannot or will I take away the pain. Instead, I encourage you to feel the pain. You cannot avoid the pain; this only intensifies the pain. Paradoxically, the only way to resolve the pain is to go through the pain. A recent encounter involved working with someone in the healing process. At one point, the release of the pain resulted in surprisingly intense sobbing session. The level of wailing can best be described by imagining a 4-year-old toddler whose wails after his/her finger has been accidentally slammed in a car door. Witnessing this from a normally stoic grown adult highlights the profound pain in the realm of sexuality. Once the pain is acknowledged and experienced, it can be transformed to something profound and healing.

There is a saying in the workout/gym/weightlifting community: No pain, no gain. Not so surprisingly, this platitude applies to healing the pain of sexuality. When this process is complete, you can experience peace and acceptance. And, you have the potential for great love.

The "Reverse-Golden-Rule."

A guideline I want to introduce as you move forward in your journey of sexual health is the "Reverse-Golden Rule." We've all heard about the Golden Rule: Treat other people as you would like to be treated. Pretty straight forward and most people get it. Have you ever heard of the "Reverse Golden Rule?" It simply states: Treat yourself the way you would treat others.

Many times in my work, clients treat themselves so poorly that I'm bothered. These individuals emotionally berate themselves, sometimes even expressing the self-hate and shame out loud. Statements such as "I'm so stupid, I'm a fuck-up, and I deserve shit" are not uncommon. When I hear this, I simply ask, "Would you treat others the way you treat yourself? Almost always, the response is No. Hence the Reverse-Golden-Rule: Treat yourself the way you would treat others. For individuals early in the sexual health journey, this is the ONLY way the person can learn self-care, self-respect, and self-love. Treating yourself with care will allow you to explore what it means to be a sexually healthy person without the shame and guilt.

How (NOT) to use this book

If you choose, you could finish this workbook in a few hours (or even less) by simply writing down quick responses to the questions. That approach, however, is not productive. This book is designed for reflection. Pay attention to the concepts of discernment and integrity. Be honest and thorough. Don't edit your responses. Simply write. If issues arise as you answer the questions, you can address them in due time. Space is available throughout the workbook, although in some cases you may need additional paper.

Life Coaching and Sexual Health

What would it look like to develop a health based, holistically integrative approach to sexuality? What would it look like if the conversation starts from a place of health versus starting from a problem? In my experience, the more enjoyable conversations occur when a person is experiencing a transformation regarding sexuality.

Often when people learn that I am a therapist, they tell me about their life. They are eager – hungry even –to share who they are with me. I've heard stories everywhere – the gym, coffee shop, walking the dogs, parties, meetings, etc. People have a real need to discover, understand, embrace and express their personal stories, perhaps as a way of gaining support. Often, however, in our society the only acceptable venue for seeking support is through the medical model of a "problem," where people seek professional help because bad things are happening.

In recent years, a "Life Coaching" movement has been developing. What is a life coach? Imagine a health-based, holistically integrative approach to self-identity, starting from a place of health, not from a problem. This growth comes from insight and understanding of your story. Life coaching uses your experiences to help you integrate your values and goals, facilitating growth. A life coach is someone who walks along in your journey toward living a life you love.

Finding a Sex Therapist

There are times, however, that professional help is needed to help an individual in his or her journey toward sexual health. I forgot the difficulty many people have in talking about sexuality. I've been in the field for 17 years at this point; sometimes it feels like all I do is talk about sex. (Is it possible to talk about sex too much?) Clients will often say, "I've never told a previous therapist about this…." and then go into a story regarding their life, sexual history, sexual behavior, or assault. I thought it might be helpful to highlight a few strategies to find a clinician who specializes in sexuality

Advocate for yourself. Check out a number of websites, including SASH.NET and AASECT.ORG. Call your insurance company for referrals to see clinicians experienced working in sexual matters.

Call. Most clinicians will take a 10-15 minute phone call to see if an initial interview should be set. Be direct and open in the phone call. This is not the time to beat around the bush. Use the time efficiently. Put your issue out there: "I'm struggling with Internet porn." "I've been sexually assaulted. Do you work with clients in this area?" "What is a summary of your treatment approach? "Do you have any resources available on the web?"

Ask for referrals. If the clinician responds no, ask him/her for referrals. Repeat the process until you have 1-3 clinicians whom you might want to meet.

Set-up a meeting. Some clinicians will have free 1/2-hour sessions, others don't. The intake interview is as much for you as it is for the clinician. Feel free to ask questions to the clinician as well. "How busy are you? What is your training/experience in this area? How many clients have you worked with on this topic?" The more forthright you will be, the more likely you will find a clinician who can help in your recovery.

Remember, the therapist is there for you, not you for the therapist.

The Importance and Limits of Confidentiality and Risk of Disclosure

Trust is a major component of counseling. Trust builds a sense of safety that leads to tremendous therapeutic change. Knowing that any information you share will not be told to others strengthens trust. In any therapeutic relationship, confidentiality limits what a professional can disclose to others. You are the one holding this privilege. Depending on where you live, however, there are limits to this privilege. Often, the limits facilitate safety in the broad sense of the term, such as requiring the professional to report any suspected abuse of a child or vulnerable adult; significant and real potential harm to yourself (e.g., if you make statements such as "I'm going to kill myself"); significant and real potential harm to another person (e.g., if you makes statements such as "I'm going to kill that person"); or when a court order requires the release of information.

As you complete the assignments, it is important to be open and honest about your past and present behaviors. While it is important for disclosure to occur, it is important for disclosure to occur in a prudent manner. Be careful when making disclosures of sexual behavior. Seriously consider whether your disclosure could trigger a mandatory report as required by the state and local laws where you live. There may be a risk of legal consequences if some of your sexual behaviors include illegal behaviors. One way to ensure privacy and confidentiality is to be specific about behaviors, but not provide any identifiable information. For example, you might want to say "Sexual partner #1" instead of giving the person's full name. It is worth repeating that the goal is to be as honest to yourself and your therapist/support network as possible, while ensuring your own safety.

Finally, consider the security of the workbook. I encourage you to write in the workbook as you progress through the assignments. Pay attention to who has access to the book and where you leave the book. It might be helpful to have a conversation with your partner about respecting your privacy.

Chapter 1: Talking About Sex

To start addressing questions of sexual health, it is important to reflect on your comfort and ability to talk about sex. I am keenly aware how difficult it is for many people to talk about sexual health issues. For many individuals, the first steps toward discussing sexual issues are shaped by shame, embarrassment, fear and guilt. I cannot stress enough how NORMAL these feelings are when opening up a new area of growth. While it is easy to say, I also know how many of these thoughts and feelings are irrational, based in cultural messages that "sex is bad," and a general aversion to addressing sexuality.

Even though these reactions are normal, I'm also aware how important it is to start the process of talking about your sexual health concerns. My experience suggests that sexuality is at the core of many of the most important aspects of our life. For many people, sexuality is the last issue to be addressed. At the same time, it is often the last issue counselors want to (and in some causes are trained to) address.

In almost every situation when someone starts the process of addressing sexuality, the reaction eventually is positive. The energy "protecting" the shame is released and redirected toward life-giving actions. New possibilities are created allowing the individual to live a new life.

I encourage people to talk about their internal process, without necessarily disclosing the content. This is where the person can share feeling statements from therapy. As an example, "I realized I felt sad …" To the degree you choose, you can add material about why you are sad.

As you move through the book, you might talk about some of the "lessons learned" from your work, without highlighting sexual health as the focus. For example, "Today's topic was on intimacy (see Chapter 9), and I realize I need to develop my skills in emotional intimacy." My experience is that, when an individual learns how to engage in these discussions, the possibility of growing in sexual health increases.

How Comfortable Are You?

The goal of this exercise is to 1) assess your ability to talk about sex and sexuality with others, and 2) identify people with whom you can talk about sex. I am confident that your comfort level will increase as you progress through your work. Below are a few ideas on how to talk about the therapy process without getting bogged down in the details of the history. The suggestions are simply a way to have a conversation with others who may be support for you.

Respond YES or NO to the following questions:

1.   I avoid talking about sex.
2.   I talk about my sexuality with my friend(s).
3.   I find many sexual matters too upsetting to talk about
4.   I talk about my sexuality with my sexual partner(s).
5.   I talk about my sexual feelings.
6.   I usually feel comfortable discussing my sexual values.
7.   I usually feel comfortable discussing topics of a sexual nature.
8.   I usually feel comfortable discussing my sexuality.
9.   Talking about sex is usually a positive experience.
10.   It bothers me to talk about sex.
11.   I usually feel comfortable discussing my sexual behavior.
12.   I feel there will be negative consequences if I talk about sex.

Score 1 point for each "NO" on questions # 2, 4–7, 9, 11. Score 1 point for each "YES" on questions # 1, 3, 8, 10, 12

Assignment

1. Reflect on the above questions: explain your responses.

2. Reflect on your thoughts and feelings as you start this journey. Many people express fear, shame, guilt and hopelessness as they look at all the topics in the workbook. How present are these thoughts and feelings?

3. Other people express feelings of hope and excitement, often because they see a pathway where none had existed previously. How present are these thoughts and feelings?

4. Having people in your life to support you in the process of improving your sexual health is important. My recommendation is you find three to five people with whom you can be totally honest. In the process of creating your personal definition of sexual health, this group will serve to counterbalance your desire to do anything you want. Name four people you could start talking to about sexuality. This list could include your pastor, your sponsor, your therapist, your friends, your colleagues, your partner/spouse or others.

5. Write one paragraph summarizing what you would like to share at this time with each person. Four simple strategies for starting the process of developing a support network include:

   a. Start small. Say, "I'm now in therapy. I need someone to support me, but I'm not ready to go into full detail right now."

b. Examine who in your life is already supportive. Expand what you might say to the person that increases your self-disclosure. You might say, "I'm working with a therapist in the area of human sexuality."

1.

2.

3.

4.

Reviewing Your Sex History

A natural progression from the exercise of talking about sex is the exercise of talking about your sexual history. As you progress toward sexual health it is important to describe accurately and completely your past sexual behavior. This document is a "living document," which means it might be helpful to return periodically to the assignment and add material as you remember pieces of your history. At first, you may not want to put everything on paper because of what others might think. You cannot treat something that's undisclosed. However, when you are open and honest, you will, in the end, have a better sense of your needs in your treatment process.

When you complete the history, please share the responses with a support person. However, at this time, I do not recommend disclosing this information to your primary partner. I do recommend that the person(s) to whom you disclose the information be trustworthy and nonjudgmental. I do support the concept of full disclosure, but that is a topic later in the book. (For your safety, please review the material on limits to confidentiality in the introduction, see page 17.)

Assignment

Complete as thoroughly as possible. Use additional paper as necessary. Update as you remember pieces of your history. For example, when used in a group format, hearing the histories of others can trigger additional memories.

Dating and Relationship Behavior

1. At what age did you begin to date or go out with girls/boys your own age?
2. Describe your level of self-confidence regarding dating.
3. How comfortable did you feel?
4. How attractive did you think you were to others?
5. If you have a same sex attraction, when did you come out to yourself? When did you come out to others?
6. Describe your dating behavior?
7. How do you meet dating partners?
8. How did your self-esteem improve or decrease as you dated more frequently?
9. Review the pattern of your relationships:
   a. Describe the number of your relationships, and the type and length of each relationship.
   b. Describe the dating/courtship that occurred in the relationship.
   c. Describe how you met these partners and how you broke up, and discuss any primary concerns you have.
   d. How quickly did sexual contact occur in the relationship?

Sexual Behavior

1. How old were you when you first had sexual intercourse?
2. How old was your partner?
3. How did you feel about the experience?
4. How many sexual partners have you had?

   Fill out a table that includes each partner, to the best of your ability.

Sample Table

Your Age	Partner's Age	Type of Sexual Contact	Where	Length of Relationship Plus Other details
16	15	Vaginal sex, oral sex	Both Parents House. Friends House.	Dated for 12 months
22	21	Vaginal sex	Hotel	1 encounter

   a. Describe what behaviors occurred. Be explicit and thorough (e.g., oral sex, vaginal sex, anal sex, mutual masturbation, kissing, touching, etc.).

   b. Describe the location (home, bedroom, public space, bathhouse, bar, etc.).

   c. What was the length of the relationship (one-night stand, occasional or casual sexual encounters that lasted a few months, longtime partnership, six-year marriage, etc.)?

   d. What percentage of all your sexual partners were one-night stands?

   e. Describe the circumstances in which you met your sexual partners.

   f. How many sexual partners of the same sex as you have you had?

      i. How did you feel about it then?

      ii. How do you feel about it now?

   g. Describe the frequency and circumstances of sexual encounters that occurred while using drugs and/or alcohol?

   h. If your number of sexual partners is too large to count, complete the assignment by examining periods of your life and estimating the number of contacts. Pick periods that make sense to you. For example:

      i. Up to age 13 (pre-adolescence), number of partners_____

      ii. Age 14–18, number of partners_____

      iii. Age 19–24, number of partners_____

      iv. First Job, number of partners_____

      v. At the time of your first significant relationship, number of partners_____

      vi. After divorce and/or end of first relationship, number of partners_____

      vii. At the time you lived at a particular address or a particular city, number of partners_____

      viii. Describe any patterns you've noticed as you complete this section.

5. Describe the frequency and circumstances of sexual contact with someone else other than your primary partner while you were married or in a committed relationship.

6. Describe any circumstances where you have intentionally avoided sexual contact with a partner or significant other. Include any underlying thoughts and feelings.

Masturbation

1. At what age did you first masturbate?
2. How did you learn about masturbation?
3. What messages did you hear about masturbation while growing up?
4. What were your beliefs and feelings about masturbation while growing up?
5. What are your beliefs and feelings about masturbating today?
6. How often do you masturbate (focus on the last 30 days)?
7. When was the last time you masturbated?
8. What thoughts and feelings did you have when you last masturbated?
9. Describe the frequency and circumstances when you masturbated somewhere other than your home?
10. When you masturbate, what objects have you used to enhance your level of sexual arousal (e.g., items of clothing, vibrators, magazines, sexual toys, items to inflict pain)? Describe the items and circumstances of their use for sexual stimulation.

Fantasy

1. Describe your three most arousing sexual fantasies.
2. How do you feel about these fantasies?
3. What messages and beliefs did you hear about having sexual fantasies?
4. What beliefs do you have about sexual fantasies today?

5. Have you ever masturbated to sexual fantasies of rape? If so, describe the fantasy, including your relationship to the victim/abuser, the frequency of the fantasy and the length of time since your last rape fantasy.

Health Concerns

1. Describe the frequency of physical problems you have experienced that affect your ability to be sexual (such as difficulties achieving or maintaining erections, difficulties having orgasms, a lack of interest in sex, difficulties in delaying ejaculation, painful penetration), and then describe the circumstances in which you experienced these difficulties.
2. Describe the frequency with which you've contracted sexually transmitted infections and the circumstances under which you were infected. How was the infection transmitted?
3. Describe any circumstances leading to pregnancy, bearing a child or being the partner of someone who became pregnant or bore a child.
4. Describe any circumstances leading to having an abortion or being the partner of someone who had an abortion.

Abuse

1. Describe the frequency of being sexually touched or being forced to engage in sexual behavior as a child. Describe the circumstances under which these instances occurred.
2. Describe the frequency of being sexually touched or being forced to engage in sexual behavior as an adult. Describe the circumstances under which these instances occurred.
3. Describe the frequency of being the target of sexual harassment, and circumstances under which these instances occurred.
4. Describe the frequency of sexual contact between you and members of your family, and describe the circumstances under which these instances occurred.
5. Describe any circumstances when you abused or sexually harassed someone else.

Children

1. Describe any sexual contact you have had with children while you were an adult.

2. Describe the content of sexually explicit pictures of children you have seen or possessed.
3. Describe the frequency of viewing explicit child sexual material and the circumstances under which you did so.
4. Have you masturbated to fantasies of sex with children? If so, describe the details.

Legal

1. Describe any legal consequences of your sexual behavior.
2. Describe the frequency of legal consequences.

Other Patterns of Sexual Behavior

1. Describe the frequency of paying money for sex or trading drugs for sex, and the circumstances under which you've done so.
2. Describe the frequency of engaging in prostitution and the circumstances under which you've done so.
3. Describe the frequency of having sexual touch with an animal, and the circumstances under which you've done so.
4. Describe the frequency of public sex, exposing your genitals to others without their consent and the circumstances under which you've done so.
5. Describe the frequency of spying on someone for sexual gratification and the circumstances under which you've done so.
6. Describe the types of sexual magazines and movies you view for sexual stimulation.
7. Describe your frequency of using threats of violence, physical force or any weapon to make someone perform a sexual act. Describe the circumstances under which you've done so.
8. Describe the frequency of participating in consensual use of restraints or consensual bondage acts, and describe the circumstances under which you've done so.
9. Describe the frequency of participating in group sex and the circumstances under which you've done so.

10. Describe the frequency of participating in alternative (culturally described as "kinky") behaviors and the circumstances under which you've done so.

Internet Related Sexual Behaviors

1. At what age did you first start using the Internet for sexual purposes? Describe the behavior and content of your first sexual online sexual experiences.

2. Describe how your frequency of using the Internet for sex changed over the years. Describe any unusual patterns.

3. Describe when you have become sexually aroused while engaging in Internet sexual behaviors. What type of activity were you involved in at the time?

4. Describe what you enjoy doing most sexually online, (e.g., looking at pornography, visiting chat rooms, exposing yourself)? How has this preference changed over time?

5. Describe the frequencies and areas of sexual activity that you enjoy exploring online, (e.g., certain ethnicities, feet, animals, diapers…).

6. Have you ever done anything sexually online that could be considered illegal? Describe in a general way.

7. Describe the frequency and circumstances when you have used virtual worlds such as Second Life to engage in virtual sex.

8. Describe the frequency and circumstances when you have used the Internet to arrange for an escort service or prostitute?

9. Describe the frequency with which you have used the Internet to meet sexual partners and the circumstances under which you used the Internet to make these connections.

10. Describe the frequency and circumstances regarding how your offline sexuality has been impacted by your online sexual behaviors?

11. Describe the frequency and circumstances regarding your posting online erotic or sexual pictures/videos of yourself or others (including via webcam or texting).

12. Describe the frequency and circumstances regarding your masturbating with online sexual materials or activities. What type of content do you typically masturbate to?

13. Describe any "ritual" you may engage in regarding your Internet sex use (e.g., planning and preparing the same way each time, cleaning/deleting files after each Internet sex session, etc.)?

14. Describe the frequency and circumstances regarding high-risk behaviors you have engaged in while online (e.g., downloading pornography at work, engaging in illegal online behaviors, etc.) What is the typical content of such materials?

15. Describe the frequency and circumstances regarding cybersex behavior which you have engaged in at work or at the houses of friends or relatives.

16. Describe the frequency and circumstances regarding physical problems resulting from your Internet sexual behavior (e.g., contracted an STD from a chat partner, been injured by a sex partner met online, etc.).

17. Describe the frequency and circumstances regarding your use of a sex toy that connects to your computer while online?

18. What other sexual activities have you engaged in while online that would be important to disclose?

General

1. Describe any sexual behaviors or practices that are not addressed in the above questions.

2. Which three questions from the section above were the most difficult to answer?
   - Why did you select these three questions?
   - What made them so difficult to answer?

3. What are three things you learned about yourself by completing this assignment?

4. Which three areas would you highlight at this time as the primary areas of concern?

Sexual Behavior Timeline

The goal of this exercise is to translate the material from your sex history into a visual format. In creating your Sexual Behavior Timeline, it possible for you to understand how your sexual behaviors have occurred across time in relation with other issues. By charting these events, you can discover patterns in your sexual behavior.

Although it is possible to see a relationship between behaviors and other issues, it is not possible to determine cause and effect. By completing the Sexual Behavior Timeline, you may get a sense of the various relationships that exist between your emotions and your sexual behavior.

Complete the following exercise as thoroughly as possible. Use the information from the previous sexual history exercise and plot the events along the horizontal timeline (see sample timeline two pages ahead), attempting to reflect on your age at the time of the event. In addition to the behaviors identified in your sexual history, plot the following life events on the time line. (See the next page for additional instructions.)

- Age when you hit puberty.

- The first time you:
    - Masturbated.
    - Masturbated at a computer.
    - Remember being attracted to another person.
    - Had an orgasm.
    - Had sex with anyone.
    - Used the Internet for sexual purposes.
    - Kept your sexual behavior hidden.
    - Felt shame regarding your sexual behavior.

- Age at relationship changes (new relationship, divorce, breakup, entering into marriage/partnership, etc.)

- Age at life changes (home move, new job, substance-abuse treatment, sobriety, first child, illness, death of a loved one, etc.).

- Any critical incidents in your life. A critical incident is any event, large or small, that has meaning in your life. (Examples: when you first self-identified as gay, the time you were sexually assaulted.).

- With color pens or pencils, track relevant behaviors. This might include tracking spending behaviors, drug or alcohol behaviors, gambling, etc. Also, track additional life events such as depression or mood changes, stress, relationship satisfaction, job satisfaction or other important events in your life, especially as they relate to your sexual behavior. Below is a simplified example to illustrate how to complete a timeline. Please feel free to adapt as necessary.

It might be helpful to tape a few pieces of paper together or use poster board to increase your space. Across the left-hand edge of the page, draw a vertical line. The vertical line should be numbered +5 to 0. At the center of the vertical line, draw a horizontal line that travels the length of the page. The horizontal line reflects your age across time. If you notice, the space on the timeline is not "equal." Some parts of your life are less relevant, so you can save space. Other times of your life may be more expansive.

You might need to devise a code to fit everything into the timeline. Some individuals have used multiple colors to chart a number of items. For some people this might be mood or chemical use or anxiety, or whatever. If, for example, at the time of a marriage you were very happy, your mood might be charted at a +5. One person charted both the amount of chemical use and mood. Afterward he was able to see the inverse relationship between mood and chemical use. The more he used, the lower his mood. Admittedly, the timeline does not necessarily show causality. His lower mood may have contributed to his increased chemical use as an attempt to self-medicate to cope with the sexual behavior.

Below the line are spaces to describe relevant events in your life. The key for the bottom part of the timeline is to examine life events and topics to see how they fit into the picture. Each timeline will be different. You are literally creating a graph of your life. What is relevant to each person varies as much as each individual. In this example, we had three items; your timeline might have more. Additional topics to graph include financial, relational, geographic and/or familial changes.

Sample Time Line

+5	
+4	Graph the intensity of important feelings
	such as grief, depression, anger, loneliness,
+3	etc. +5 very intense, 0 Not present.
+2	
+1	
0	

Write out the major components of your sex history along this line

Include major life events in your life. It is helpful to write small.

Age	10	18	19	24	30
Relevant Life History Info	Parents divorced	College	Failed out of college	First serious relationship	Broke up
Sexual Behavior History	Saw porn for the first time on the Internet	Porn use increased both in time and graphic, content	Looking at porn and masturbating for more than 8 hours a day	Great sex life Happy	Internet
Chemical History Info		Binge drinking	Begin using pot. Hooked up with meth. First treatment	In recovery	Relapsed

Reflect on your timeline, identify three insights you learned.

1.

2.

3.

Chapter 2: Culture, Values and Stereotypes

Power of Thought

A lot of emphasis in this workbook focuses on helping you understand your thinking patterns. To do so, we first need to discuss the power of thought.[2] The basic premise is that all aspects of our entire existence are based on thought – that thought shapes how we perceive and examine life events, our feelings, and our interactions with others. These thoughts are linked together and become a story (see, Power of Story, page 2). This section discusses why I believe thought is so powerful.

At one point in the Broadway musical *Wicked*, the heroine enters Oz, where the citizens wear green-colored glasses. Over time, the citizens had forgotten they were wearing green glasses, and simply concluded that everything was in fact green. This was why Oz appeared to be an "Emerald City." In a similar way, our thinking patterns color our view of life. These patterns are so pervasive that we simply don't realize they are present. Sometimes the assumptions have a limited impact in our lives; other times, these thinking patterns are so unhealthy they result in painful consequences. In many ways, the cultures we belong to are the lenses we use to look at the world. Our awareness of these lenses has disappeared simply because we see through them versus seeing them. Moving toward sexual health means moving toward understanding the cultural lenses we use to understand the world.

Our cultural views shape both our worldview and our experience of each moment. Within each moment our awareness and knowledge are based on perceptions, and through the almost instantaneous analysis of these perceptions, we arrive at a conclusion (i.e., a "thought") that guides our feelings, choices and behaviors. This is a bit different from conventional wisdom, which often dictates that feelings come first. Yet, consider the following scenarios:

You parked your car on the street. As you return from the store, you find your car is gone. The awareness is that your car is missing. The feelings result from the conclusions based on various thoughts. Depending on the thought, your feelings might be different. Consider the following:

> You have been reading the newspaper about stolen cars in the neighborhood. The thought that percolates to your awareness is, "My car has been stolen," and you probably have feelings of anger or of being violated, or both.

> As an alternative, you notice a "No Parking" sign during high traffic/rush hours. You happen to have parked your car just before that time began, and you returned to find you car gone. Your thought might be, "My car has been towed." Notice, however, your feelings are different based on your thoughts. You might feel anger, embarrassment, frustration or shame because you feel you should have known better.

> Consider a third possibility. You're talking on a cell phone, as you get to where you thought you parked your car, you realize it is gone. You think, "My car is gone" with thoughts of anger, violation, frustration, etc. Then you notice that six spaces up is your car. Because you were distracted, you went to the wrong space. The corresponding feelings might be embarrassment, relief, and/or humor as you realize how you overreacted.

These three examples help explain how thoughts shape your feelings and subsequent behaviors. One author highlights how much of our thought is actually automatic and can occur in the blink of an eye[3]. Sometimes we simply don't realize how many different thoughts we have in a particular moment. Not true, you say? Think about how many complicated tasks, thoughts and attention to stimuli occur while you drive a car. Yet, you never *think* about driving a car. You simply drive.

Two strategies to use at this point for increasing the awareness of the power of your thoughts are "mindfulness" and "transference." Both are powerful tools that give us insight into the power of thought.

Mindfulness

Mindfulness is the experience of being aware of your current thoughts, feelings, body state and surroundings by paying attention to your reactions, motivations and actions. To increase your ability to be mindful, I encourage you to become aware of your inner conversation. When someone walks into the room, we may say to the person next to us, "She's attractive." But our inner conversation is what we have with ourselves when no one is around. Someone might walk into the room, and we say to ourselves, "I want to have sex with her." Various meditation techniques can also be helpful in increasing your mindfulness.

Transference

Transference is any reaction we have to another person. Often the experience of transference occurs so quickly, we don't realize either that it occurred or the content of the transference. We are CONSTANTLY assessing and judging our environment based on our past experience. This is a NORMAL part of life. It is how we process many of daily experiences simply because there is too much material to process. It is the past experience applied to the current situation that typifies transference. Most of the time we focus on negative transference, or the negative reactions we have to someone, but positive transference is also helpful to understand. In any reaction, you can learn what you are feeling and thinking and how it relates to your acting-out cycle. The individuals with whom we have the strongest reaction are perhaps the people who can teach us the most. It is your reaction that tells you the most about yourself. Ask yourself the following questions: "Why am I having this reaction? Who does this remind me of? What memory does this person trigger? Why do I like or dislike this person?" Whatever the response, you can gain insight into your internal thoughts and feelings. The key is that your reaction is about you.

Taken together, mindfulness and transference are two important concepts to help you increase your awareness of your thoughts. Much of what we think occurs so automatically that we see the picture but fail to see the pieces of the puzzle.

- Mindfulness is the process of becoming aware of the "here and now." Start to increase your awareness of your current thoughts.

- If any emotional reaction, identify the thoughts associated with the reaction.

- Describe the underlying thought relating to any experience of transference.

- Start to examine patterns of thinking related to sexuality that appear to be present in your life. What themes appear to be present at this point?

Culture and Stereotypes

You are a product of the multiple cultures to which you belong (such as racial, ethnic, religious and age), and these cultures are sometimes in harmony and other times in a tug-of-war. In this section, we look at a variety of cultures as they shape our lives. We examine the cultures to which you might belong, and we also take a special look at the culture and components of sexual identity.

Your Cultures and Stereotypes

Everything we know is taught to us through cultures. Much of what we see as sexually arousing is defined by the cultures to which we belong — such as family, race, gender, religious connection, sexual identity or nationality — and the things that sexually arouse us can change over time. These cultures shape sexual behaviors, values and identity. Improving your sexual health requires that you increase your awareness of your cultural values. It is important for you to understand all of the cultures to which you belong and how they influence your thoughts, beliefs and expectations. Shorthand ways of understanding the world are labeled as stereotypes. The discussion is designed to help you identify and challenge some stereotypes

Most of the time, we simply exist within our cultures without any difficulties. Sometimes, however, the various cultures to which we belong may conflict with one another. For example, in Latino culture, "machismo" (loosely understood as hypermasculinity) is a typical male stereotype, and it is considered wrong for a man to show any weakness or feminine characteristics. If a man who belongs to the Latino culture wants to acknowledge that he is attracted to other men, then the two cultures are in conflict. Resolving such conflicts is crucial to increasing your personal sexual health. Some people resolve such conflicts by rejecting parts of their heritage; others work toward changing the culture they came from. They key is for you to integrate the cultures to which you belong within your overall identity.

Assignment

Identify the various cultures to which you belong. Identify two sexual beliefs you learned from each culture. Consider the following types of cultures:

Racial Culture

Racial Culture is often used synonymously with "skin color." (This usage is limiting, but I use it here for our general discussion.) It is important to see how your thoughts are shaped by assumptions about race.

Please complete the following sentences:

I belong to the_____ racial culture. Two sexual beliefs I learned are:

1.

2.

Ethnic / Nationality Culture

For our purposes, I use this term to describe national origin. Are you from Poland, Indonesia, or Senegal? Some ethnic cultures cross over national boundaries. And many countries have multiple ethnic groups.

Please complete the following sentences:

I belong to the_____ culture. Two sexual beliefs I learned are:

1.

2.

Religious Culture

This refers to the shared beliefs regarding God and spirituality. In the United States, these beliefs might include (among others) Judeo-Christian, Islamic or Atheistic beliefs, but even within each religious tradition are multiple sub-cultures that shape sexual values.

Please complete the following sentences:

I belong to the_____ culture. Two sexual beliefs I learned are:

1.

2.

Age

The era in which we grew up and the generation to which we belong influence our sexual views. Someone who grew up in the 1930's views sexuality differently from someone who grew up in the 1970's. This results in different values that shape sexuality.

Please complete the following sentences:

I belong to the_____ culture. Two sexual beliefs I learned are:

1.

2.

Gender and Sexual Orientation

We'll look at sexual identity in detail (see page 47) but for now, let's say sexual identity includes our gender (male/female), and sexual orientation (gay/straight/bi). There are numerous stereotypes regarding sexual identity. Each stereotype shapes our understanding of sexuality.

Please complete the following sentences:

I belong to the (male/female/trans)_____ culture. Two sexual beliefs I learned are:

1.

2.

I identify as (gay/bi/straight)_____. Two sexual beliefs I learned are:

1.

2.

Socioeconomic Status

Socioeconomic status means your level of wealth and your standard of living. Socio-economic status shapes your view of sexuality. (For example, sharing a bed with a parent takes on a new meaning if you have a one-room house.) Please complete the following sentences, indicating whether you belong to a wealthy, middle class or poor socioeconomic culture.

Please complete the following sentences:

I belong to the_____ culture. Two sexual beliefs I learned are:

1.

2.

Disability Status

Disability refers to mental, physical, or emotional disabilities. Some may occur at birth (mental handicap), or be acquired (illnesses). There are beliefs based on disability.

Please complete the following sentences:

I belong to the (disabled_____) (non-disabled_____) culture. Two sexual beliefs I learned are:

1.

2.

Geographic Status

Geographic status can be national or regional. Within the United States, for example, there are differences in sexual values based on region – northern, southern, eastern, and western. Please complete the following sentences:

I belong to the_____ culture.

Two sexual beliefs I learned are:

1.

2.

Online Cyber Culture

This refers to the thoughts you have about online sexual behaviors.

Please complete the following sentences:

Two sexual beliefs I learned are:

1.

2.

After reviewing your answers, think about what you've learned about yourself or others based on this assignment. How have these beliefs shaped your sexual behavior? Share with your support team. Be sure to challenge some of the assumptions you listed.

- Which cultural messages are unhelpful to you?

- Which cultural messages are helpful to you?

- Each of us is a product of the many cultures to which we belong. What values from different cultures are in conflict? How do you resolve such conflicts?

Feelings of Shame and Guilt

By definition, culture is where we learn shame and guilt. Many people struggle with shaming messages about sexuality. It is important to understand the difference between the two. Below we highlight our understanding of the basic differences between shame and guilt. Consider how shame and guilt relate to your sexual behavior.

Shame

Shame is a feeling based on a thought that as a person, you are bad, worthless, unforgiveable, and defective. Shame is *person focused*. ("I am a bad person.") The associated thought is that everyone knows and rejects you. There is a belief that nothing can fix the shame, that you will never be able to get better, or that you cannot find redemption. Associated feelings of shame are despair, hopelessness, loneliness, embarrassment and humiliation. When people have feelings of shame, their behaviors often hurt both themselves and others. Shame-based behaviors can include a lack of respect for themselves and others, justification for abuse toward themselves and others and lack of empathy for others. Often shame exists within a cognitive framework of perfectionism ("I can't make a mistake; it has to be perfect. All sexual material is bad."). People who feel shame often focus on covering up, hiding and displaying a false front to mask their intense feelings. Because of shame, people will engage in behaviors to compensate in the hope that others will like them. People who feel shame lose a sense of boundaries in an attempt to cope. Some writers distinguish between healthy and toxic shame. [4] I believe that all shame is unhealthy, and that a person needs to distinguish between shame and guilt.

Guilt

Guilt is a feeling based on a thought that your behavior is wrong, bad, awful, terrible and hurtful. Guilt is the recognition that you violated your ethical values and morality. Guilt is *act focused*. ("I feel guilty when I have done something wrong.") When you feel guilty about something you have done, you do not have to feel shame. Because guilt is about your behavior, you usually can do something about it. You can apologize, forgive, learn, change, develop and grow in response to the guilt. You can set boundaries, repair the damage and rebuild relationships. Guilt is normal, appropriate and even healthy. Guilt is unhealthy when you feel an inappropriate amount of guilt, or when you feel guilty when you haven't done anything wrong. If these feelings are present, you are probably stuck in shame. I encourage you to feel guilty when the feeling is appropriate. In the context of sexual health, some behaviors are wrong and guilt is the recognition that you did something wrong (e.g., "I lied about what I did").

You learn both shame and guilt from the same sources, including family of origin, religion, school, friends, government, and society. Learning the concept of responsibility is also a cultural process. A person learns responsibility through parenting, role modeling and holding others accountable for their behavior. The goal for individuals is to learn from their mistakes. In our society, shame is taught more often than responsibility. The phrase, "*Shame on you*" should be changed to "*Guilt on you*."

It is important to examine cultural sources of shame such as racism, sexism and heterosexism. Each of these forms of prejudice shows a negative judgment on entire groups. From these cultural sources of shame, individuals learn shame directly (overt) and indirectly (covert). Individuals are taught that being different is wrong. Shame is taught overtly when children are told they are bad, they're put down as worthless, or they're made fun of and teased cruelly. People who violate the boundaries of others in emotional, psychological, physical and sexual ways teach shame. Covert shaming (such as a negative comments made about gay people in news media) can be difficult to recognize. It is based in poor education, poor modeling and unsupportive relationships.

Assignment

One assignment I sometimes give individuals who are stuck in shame is to list 100, or even 500, shaming messages they tell themselves. They will often resist, but once the start they are amazed at how easy it is to identify the messages. The second part of the assignment is to challenge the underlying thinking errors that contribute to the shaming messages. Ask yourself the following questions:

• What shameful messages did you hear growing up?

• Who provided these messages?

• How do these messages impact you today?

• What shaming messages did you hear regarding sexuality?

• If part of a minority group (e.g., you're a woman, a person of color, a gay person, etc.), what shaming messages have you heard?

- What shaming messages do you experience now?

- What sexual behaviors trigger feelings of shame?

- Now, repeat the same questions substituting the word *shame* with the word *guilt*.

Sexual Identity and Sexual Orientation

The next section discusses the process of forming sexual identity and sexual orientation and the related tasks. People use the two terms interchangeably, but they are in fact different. All messages of sexual identity are culturally informed. It is important to review how your sexual identity relates to your sexual health.

Sexual Identity Development for All

Identity is a statement "this is who I am." In the process of clarifying this identity, individuals go through a process of sorting through life events, responding "like-me/not like me." This is an oversimplification, but identity development is the attempt to define and understand who we are. It is an interactive process that everyone goes through – often unconsciously in understanding their sexual selves. Obviously, this process also occurs in the area of sexual identity.

Four Components of Sexual Identity

Sexual identity is complex. Following are four components of sexual identity. Each component plays a role in your sexual identity.

Natal Sex

This refers to your biological makeup at birth. Often this refers to your sexual genitalia or your DNA makeup. Women have X-X chromosomes, while men have X-Y chromosomes. Most often this correlates to vaginal or penile genitalia.[5] Most of the time, identifying a person's genital sex is as simple as observing the baby when it's born. ("It's a *boy*!" or "It's a *girl*!")

Gender Identity

Gender Identity is the gender you feel you are. Most often this matches one's natal sex. "I have the genitalia of a female, and I feel female." When natal sex does not match Gender Identity (i.e., it is not congruent), the situation falls under the broad term "transgender." People who are transgender believe they are the opposite sex from their physical body. People described that they feel trapped in the wrong body. For example, a biological male believes he is female, or a biological female believes she is male. Identifying as transgender is not a psychosis or neurosis. If you believe that you are transgender, please seek help from a trained professional. It is a complex topic beyond the scope of this workbook.

Social Sex Roles

Easy to understand but often misunderstood, social sex roles refer to culturally defined behaviors based on one's gender. Typically, social sex roles are divided into masculine roles and feminine roles, but these roles may change over time, hence the potential for confusion. Social sex roles reflect what a man is "supposed to be like" or what a woman is "supposed to be like." Often, social sex roles are confused with sexual identity – for example, an effeminate male labeled as "gay." Common thoughts such as "All guys do it" or "Women aren't sexual" are thinking errors related to social sex roles. These are examples of how culture shapes our social sex roles.

Sexual Orientation

This is most often described as a same-sex attraction or a heterosexual attraction. Often people simply say, "I'm a gay man" or "I'm a lesbian woman" or "I'm a straight female." This concept is not necessarily clear-cut.

Assignment

Review the four components of sexual identity. Complete the following.

- Natal Sex: I identify as _____.

- Gender Identity: I identify as _____.

- Social Sex Roles: Describe 3-4 social sex roles reflecting your gender identity. What does it mean for you to be (insert gender identity here:) _____.

Sexual Orientation Explored

In the pre-Internet days, if a person wanted to gain information on sexual orientation, the few places to look were typically a dictionary or an encyclopedia article. For many, the fear of asking a librarian for help was too much. Now, the Internet makes such information easily available. Much research has gone into understanding the causes of sexual orientation. Generally, the conclusion is that science just does not know.

No single scientific theory about what causes sexual orientation has been suitably substantiated. Studies to associate sexual orientation with genetic, hormonal, and environmental factors have so far been inconclusive. Sexual orientation is no longer considered to be one's conscious individual preference or choice, but is instead thought to be formed by a complicated network of social, cultural, biological, economic, and political factors. *Sex Information and Educational Council of the US (SIECUS), 1993.*

There are a number of myths regarding the cause of a same-sex attraction. The research makes it clear that a history of sexual abuse does not cause a same-sex attraction. Same-sex orientation is not a psychopathology. Based on research showing no greater evidence of mental illness among individuals with same-sex attractions vs. those with an opposite-sex attraction, in 1973, the American Psychiatric Association removed homosexuality from its list of mental health disorders. An individual's sexual orientation also appears to stabilize over time. What might change, however, is one's acceptance of, or expression of, one's sexual orientation. All major health associations in the United States, including the American Psychiatric Association, the American Medical Association and the American Psychological Association, consider it unethical to attempt to change one's sexual orientation (known as the ex-gay movement or reparative therapy).

The "Kinsey Continuum" was an early attempt to understand sexual orientation and sought to rate one's *genital sexual behaviors* on a scale ranging from "exclusively heterosexual" to "exclusively homosexual." Adaptations of the continuum include "fantasy content" and "emotional relationships." Look at each topic to see where you fit on the continuum. With whom do you have sexual contact? What gender is in your fantasies? Who are your closest friends?

Adapted Kinsey Continuum

0	1	2	3	4	5	6
Exclusively Opposite Sex						Exclusively Same Sex

Stages of Identity Development

Many people who have a same-sex identity experience a process of moving toward a place of acceptance. We call this a "coming out process." Vivian Cass presents one model of identity development that might be helpful in understanding a same-sex sexual identity. She hypothesizes six stages:

Stage 1 — Identity Confusion

Heterosexual identity is called into question with a person's increasing awareness of feelings of intimate and physical attraction toward others of the same sex. Individuals will start asking themselves the question "Could I be homosexual?" Gay and lesbian information or awareness on the Internet becomes personally relevant, and the heterosexual assumption begins to be undermined.

Stage 2 — Identity Comparison

Individuals begin accepting the potential that homosexual feelings are a part of the self. The realization that "I might be homosexual" may cross your mind. Perhaps due to shame and guilt, the individual expresses a same-sex identity only online. The idea that "I may be bisexual" (which permits the potential for heterosexuality) can also be a manifestation of this stage. It is also at this level that the belief "This is a 'phase' I'm going through" may surface. These strategies reduce the incongruence between same-sex attractions and a view of one's self as heterosexual. The task at this stage of identity comparison, according to Cass, is to deal with social alienation as the individual becomes aware the individual's difference from larger society.

Stage 3 — Identity Tolerance

This is marked by statements such as, "I only look at gay stuff online, but I don't do anything with other people." Online behaviors may be a tool used at this stage. This declaration results in a sense of clarity for individuals, but it also results in a sense of separation from others, because the individuals recognize that they are "different." For individuals who experience a heightened need for peer approval and acceptance, this can be a difficult period. During this period, individuals often create a well-developed facade to "mask" and hide this part of them. Individuals often struggle with a constant need to hide their sexual orientation. Positive experiences are crucial to developing a degree of self-acceptance during this period. Contacting other gay, lesbian and/or bisexual people becomes a more pressing issue to alleviate a sense of isolation and alienation. It also provides individuals with the experience of accepting their whole being.

Stage 4 — Identity Acceptance

Contact with other gays and lesbians is important and increases. Although this was difficult for older generations, younger generations are often easily able to find support groups. Those individuals fortunate enough to have access to support groups or social events often experience a heightened sense of their identity and a sense of self-acceptance. There is a move away from hiding the identity to sharing their identity with people in their life.

Stages 5 and 6 — Identity Pride and Identity Synthesis

Individuals move from a "them and us" mentality into a realization and acceptance of the similarities between the heterosexual and homosexual worlds. Strong identification with the gay subculture and devaluation of heterosexuality and many of its institutions (Stage 5) give way to less rigid, polarizing views and more inclusive and cooperative behavior (Stage 6).

Men Who Have Sex with Men: Not All Gay-Sex is Gay

Not all men who have sex with men will identify as being gay. In many cases, we use the phrase "men who have sex with men" to focus on the behavior versus a label. Some of these men do not identify as gay because they are "in the closet" and in denial about their sexual orientation, attempting to minimize, avoid or deny their same-sex attractions. In some cases, men who have sex with men are truly not gay. For these men, having sex with another man results in minimal guilt, because they can say "I didn't have sex with another woman" or because it supports the flattering notion that they can find sexual partners easily. In some situations (prison, military or religious settings), the only available sexual partner is someone of the same gender (a/k/a "situational homosexuality"). For this person, if both genders were available, he would choose the opposite gender. As a final example, the behavior may have occurred under the influence of alcohol or other chemicals.

While all of these examples show men engaging in sexual behavior with people of the same sex, their behaviors do not add up to a "gay identity." A great resource on this issue is at http://www.straightguise.com/ Joe Kort has identified 12 types of same-sex behavior that may not be the result of a gay-identity. Unfortunately, there is limited similar research paralleling female same-sex behavior.

Bisexuality

In my opinion, bisexuality (a sexual orientation where a person is attracted to both men and women) is a true orientation. What makes understanding bisexuality difficult is that it is sometimes used to describe a transitory term in the coming-out process. This multiple uses of the term leads to confusion in the larger community that can make it harder for a person to clarify a bisexual orientation. A bisexual person has to cope with stereotypes from the straight community and also from the gay and lesbian communities. It is sometimes said that a bisexual has to "come out" twice, once in the straight community and a second time in the gay/lesbian community. As you examine your sexual identity, consider whether a bisexual orientation is related to your sexual behavior.

Often, people think bisexuality is only about sex, but there are many variables to consider. Regarding sexual orientation, there are three variables: genital behavior, physical attraction, and emotional attraction. For instance, think about whom you connect with emotionally. Think about whom you are attracted to intellectually or socially. You might realize, "I may be attracted to men on a physical level, but I connect better with women on an emotional level." In thinking about these variables, you get the idea that whether someone is bisexual will depend on how you ask the question.

Assignment

- Using the Kinsey Scale (described 3 pages above) how would you describe your sexual orientation?

- Review your sexual history. How many partners were of the same sex as you?

- What positive, negative or shameful messages have you heard about the four components of sexual identity (Natal Sex, Gender Identity, Social Sex Roles, Sexual Orientation) related to your personal experience. How have these affected your sexual health?

Chapter 3: Physical Components of Sexual Health

One of the easier aspects for both individuals and professionals to address is the physical or bodily aspect of sexual health. In the research literature, MOST of the research focuses on these aspects. Sexual Health is often described as a medical issue, and focuses on functioning concerns. Another focus of physical health is disease prevention regarding sexually transmitted illnesses (STI) and HIV. Much of the recent progress in sexual health promotion in the last 15 to 25 years is paradoxically a response to HIV and a public discussion regarding sexuality. This chapter briefly examines at a number of physical aspects of sexual health including sexual functioning, sexual dysfunction, health care and safer sex concerns regarding STI/HIV and pregnancy.

What is Sexual Functioning

Sexual health is not merely the avoidance of unhealthy behaviors. It is also the ability and confidence to engage successfully in healthy sexual behaviors. Such ability is defined as sexual functioning. The goal of this section is for you to address your level of sexual functioning, enabling you to examine the relationship between your sexual behaviors and your sexual functioning, spot issues and develop plans for addressing those issues.

Depending on the cause, there are three potential approaches for treating sexual functioning issues: (1) treating physical health (e.g., getting a physical), (2) treating symptoms (e.g., communication/relaxation) and (3) learning techniques/skills (e.g., performing Kegel exercises, sensation focusing).

A complete medical check-up is the starting point for intervention in cases of sexual dysfunction. If there is a medical condition, no amount of talk therapy will help. (This demonstrates the importance of being able to talk about sex and sexuality. See, Talking About Sex, page 19.) Your doctor might not raise the issue, so be prepared to mention it yourself. If the medical examination eliminates physical concerns, then the source of the problem might be a mental health concern (see page 72). Finally, sometimes the intervention may simply be educational. For example, some men do not know how to stimulate the woman's clitoris to help her reach orgasm. That is an example of sexual dysfunction eliminated through discovery and education.

Respond YES or NO to the following statements:

1.   I feel pressured to have sex by my sexual partner(s).

   [ ] Check here if no current sexual partner.

2.   I avoid sex because of problems with sexual functioning.

3.   I do not find sex pleasurable.

4.   Most of the time, I reach orgasm ("come") too quickly when I am with my partner(s).

5.   I have concerns about my sexual functioning.

6.   FOR MEN: I have trouble getting or keeping an erection.

   FOR WOMEN: I have trouble with lubrication (getting wet).

7.   I think I might have a sexual functioning problem caused by a medical condition or prescription medications.

8.   I often have a delay or absence of orgasm when I am with a sexual partner.

9.   I have physical pain during sexual intercourse.

10.   I usually am able to reach orgasm ("come") when I am with my partner(s).

11.   I think I might have a sexual functioning problem caused by drinking or using illegal drugs.

12.   I have no interest in having sex.

13.   I am generally satisfied with my sexual behavior.

14.   I feel anxious about my ability to perform sexually.

15.   I often have a delay or absence of orgasm when I masturbate.

16.   I have no interest in having sexual intercourse.

17.   FOR MEN: I gave myself a testicular exam in the last 30 days.

   FOR WOMEN: I gave myself a breast exam in the last 30 days.

Any "yes" response to statements 1–9, 11–12, and 14–16 require further investigation. Any "no" response to statements 10, 13, and 17 require further investigation.

The majority of sexual functioning issues include:

General Types of Sexual Dysfunction Issues

The following descriptions of dysfunction are broad and are not intended to address specifics necessary to address particular cases. It is a place for you to start a conversation with your support network.

Problems achieving orgasm

Problems achieving orgasm occur in men and women, yet women experience it more often. Treatment might not be physical and may require medical review. Sometimes, a women's partner needs education to assist her in achieving orgasm. Side effects of some medications can affect desire and interfere with orgasm. Sexual desire changes over time. Decreased sexual desire is normal in some situations (e.g., as we age). Sometimes, however, it is not normal, such as when caused by medical issues (e.g., hormonal changes or mental health issues). Sexual Aversion is an extreme avoidance or negative reaction to sexuality or sexual behavior. Usually, this is a mental health issue.

Female Physical Dysfunction Issues

Dyspareunia and *Vaginismus* are issues affecting female genitalia. The primary experience is pain in the genital area, usually during penetration. The causes vary, and medical review is required for diagnosis and treatment. Although the majority of causes are medical, psychological issues (such as unresolved abuse issues) can contribute to these conditions.

Male Physical Dysfunction Issues

Male dysfunction issues are categorized as impotence problems and ejaculation problems (premature and retarded). Get a medical check-up to eliminate physical causes, and ask your physician to address any sexual functioning concerns based on biomedical causes or medications. If physical, biomedical and medication-related causes are ruled out, then you should consult a trained therapist. Your particular problem will require a custom tailored intervention. Also, consider what parts of the process in the next section need to be addressed.

Assignment

- Review and update your sexual history and timeline when have you experienced sexual functioning issues? If any, your plans to address these are:

- Have there been changes in your sexual behavior because of functioning concerns (increased online behaviors, increased masturbation, avoidance of sex, or use of sexually explicit material because of problems with erections or painful penetration)?

- Describe any times where you had pain when engaging in sexual behavior? If any, your plans to address these are as follows:

- Are any mental health concerns related to sexual functioning?

- Medication changes or chemical use can adversely affect your sexual functioning. Are any of these relevant?

- If sexual functioning concerns are present, what are your plans to address the issues?

- What questions do you have about sexual anatomy and functioning?

- As you age, what concerns do you have regarding sexual functioning?

Treatments for sexual dysfunction vary. It is impossible to list all possible treatment approaches for sexual dysfunction because they need to be tailored to the individual. The basic approaches address physical health issues, address the symptoms, develop skills (e.g., communication/relaxation), or work on techniques (e.g., Kegel exercises, sensation focus). Please work with a clinician trained in this area if this is a problem.

Sexual Functioning and Development of Sexual Skills

People view a typical sexually explicit movie or Internet pornography and they assume – unrealistically - that they need to have sex "like a porn star." The performance expectations created have to be challenged. Real people do not perform sexually the way suggested in pornography. In addition, many individuals struggle with so much sexual shame that they simply shut down any sexual energy. Individuals struggling with sexual anorexia/sexual avoidance may believe they lack the skills needed to engage in sex. For individuals struggling with sexual anxiety, sex evokes such anxiety that it results in unpleasant experiences, creating a never-ending cycle leading to additional anxiety. Sexually compulsive individuals sometimes focus on one type of sexual experience at the expense of all other types of sexual intimacy. One goal of sexual health is the development of the knowledge, comfort, and skills for engaging in a variety of forms of sexual expression.

Sexual Health requires self-knowledge, and the awareness to assertively communicate what you want. Some individuals look for a particular type of sexual intimacy, but they don't know how to ask for it. Or – if they do know how to ask for what they are seeking – they don't know how to maintain that intimacy. Often, the individual and the partner don't feel comfortable talking about the different types of sexual intimacy. From the cybersex world, sometimes, the lack of sexual contact in real time is both a cause – and a result - of online sexual behavior.

As part of the process of addressing sexual functioning issues, exercises exist to help you develop the skills in a step-by-step process, moving toward increasingly complex skills.

Assignment

Following this paragraph is a list of different types of sexual intimacy ranked in increasing levels of intensity. Consider each step. (This process can take months.) Some steps may be easier than others. It is important to develop and maintain open communication with your partner. Your partner's willingness to participate is crucial; this may require couples therapy. Obviously if you are struggling with intimacy issues, quickies or one-time encounters may interfere with your healing. The key is to move slowly. When you feel anxiety or discomfort, say so, slow down and, if necessary, stop. Comfort at each level is necessary before moving to the next step. After each experience, reflect on and talk about your experience. Doing so will give you insight into what was easy and liked, or difficult and disliked, and ultimately whether you think you are ready to move toward the next step. If something is too uncomfortable or too anxiety producing, you may have to stay at that step for a while, or even return to an earlier step.

Types of Sexual Intimacies

Looking. The place to start is awareness of attraction. What kind of person do you find attractive? What characteristics do you like? Not like? Focus beyond just the physical and include aspects of how the other person talks with you and treats you. What are the other person's values regarding sexuality? Share your responses with your support system. Provide them with examples. Recognizing your attractions leads to the next step.

Flirting. The next step is disclosure to the person to whom you are attracted. Often this is where people get stopped. This step requires addressing fears of rejection. In some cases, rather than dealing with rejection, people either shut down their attractions or settle for someone else.

Spending time together. Learning how to spend time together is the next step. Sometimes this may be simply going out to coffee or dinner, or a more formal type of date. Review the discussion on dating (starting on page 167). Dating typically means spending time together.

Touching. Learning healthy, safe and respectful touch is a next step. This can involve simply holding hands, perhaps dancing or even light kissing. Being able to express what you like and don't like is a part of this process. At this part of the development, the assumption is that you are "clothes on." Future steps will introduce the experience of clothes off. At this point, the goal is to simply be comfortable with touch.

Kissing and Petting. At this step, you move toward increased physical touch. It is assumed that the clothes are still on, and that the touch focuses on areas other then genitalia and breasts. You might focus on touching parts of the face, hands, head, etc. As with all other steps, it is important to be aware of what you like/dislike and what feels comfortable/uncomfortable. Ongoing communication with your partner and support system is also assumed.

Nurturing and Full Body Touch. In this stage, you still have your clothes on, but the level of touch has increased to the point where multiple parts of the body are touching. You may also be sitting next to each other on a couch, etc., or lying next to each other. This level of touch is sometimes described as "spooning" or laying front to back. As with the previous two steps, starting with touching non-genital parts of the body, moving toward eventual touching the genitals/breasts over the clothes. This part of the process is deeply connected to your image of your body and genitals (see page 93).

Nudity. The next level is being next to each other naked. This may have to start slowly, for example, simply being in undergarments before being naked. Again, it is important to start off touching parts of the body other than breasts and genitalia. Once the touch is comfortable, move toward touching your partner's genitalia.

Masturbation and Mutual Masturbation. Continuing up the scale of intensity, the next step is masturbating yourself in front of your partner and watching your partner masturbate. Many individuals struggle with shame, guilt, and embarrassment around masturbation. Reviewing the discussion on masturbation (see page 98) may be helpful to help you increase self-awareness on this issue. Mutual masturbation (you masturbating your partner and your partner masturbating you) is the next step. At this point, orgasm isn't the goal, simply being comfortable with the level of touch and sexual intimacy is the key. Your level of arousal will ebb and flow, even within the encounter. The goals are being comfortable with your body and being with your partner without expectations. Identify which parts of your body lead to the highest level of arousal and share this information with your partner (i.e., your hot spots!). Perhaps when you are comfortable with the touch, orgasm through masturbation can be introduced at this level. Orgasm may also be introduced at the later stages as well.

Fantasy. Fantasies are extremely powerful. They are far up the scale because they give others a view of the innermost part of the person. It takes a lot of trust to share your fantasy with your partner. Reviewing the discussion on fantasy (see page 101) and discussing your fantasies with your therapist may be helpful before sharing your fantasy with your partner.

Penetration. The next step is developing comfort with sexual intercourse. The first step at this point is feeling comfortable with penetration. Understanding what you like/dislike, and what feels comfortable/uncomfortable is the key. Learning strategies and positions for penetration are required as well. Some people struggle with penetration due to pain, shame, or fear. As with all stages, reflection and conversation with your support system and your partner is important.

Orgasm. Clinicians disagree whether orgasm is required in the final stage. Many individuals do see it as the goal and they struggle with experiencing an orgasm. Too often, we assume orgasm has to be like the images we see in sexually explicit material, either online or videos. And, obviously, orgasm feels great. Orgasm isn't always required or needed. It is included, however, because my goal is to help you develop the skills, comfort, and self-awareness to experience orgasm. At this step, all of what you learned in the previous steps is used to facilitate success at this step. It is difficult to provide universal instructions, so working with your support system and your partner is very important.

Assignment

- Consult with your medical doctor to address any sexual functioning concerns that are based on *medical* causes.

- If you still experience sexual functioning concerns that are not based on medical causes, consider what parts of the above process you need to address? What do you need to discuss with your partner?

- Develop a plan to build your sexual experience and skills.

Safer-Sex Issues

Respond YES or NO to the following statements:

1. I feel too embarrassed to buy condoms.
2. I fear getting HIV/AIDS or another sexually transmitted infection.
3. It is my responsibility to use a condom with my sexual partner(s).
4. I would use condoms if my partner asked me.
5. Condoms are embarrassing to use.
6. I want information on feeling better about my sexuality.
7. I have had anal or vaginal sexual intercourse without a condom in the last 30 days.
8. I feel I am at high risk for getting HIV/AIDS or another sexually transmitted infection.
9. I worry I might be infected with a sexually transmitted infection.
10. I want information on sexually transmitted infections.
11. I feel ashamed when seeking medical care for sexually transmitted infections.
12. I feel comfortable when I touch my genitals.
13. Condoms make sex less pleasurable.
14. I have noticed physical genital change in the last 30 days that concern me.
15. My partner would use condoms if I asked him/her.
16. I want information on how to practice safer sex.
17. I worry that I might be infected with HIV.
    [ ] check here if you know you are HIV+.
18. I want information on HIV/AIDS.
19. I know how to use a condom correctly.
20. I engaged in unsafe sexual behavior in the last 30 days.

Score 1 point for each "yes" response to the following statements: 1–2, 5–7, 8–11, 13–14, 16–18, 20. Score 1 point for each "no" response to the following statements: 3, 4, 12, 15, 19. The higher the score, the increased risk to your overall sexual health and HIV/STI.

The questions above reflect research into the relationship between sexual health and safer-sex concerns that underlie increased risk for HIV transmission and sexually transmitted infection (STIs). They also reflect areas of focus in your progress toward improved sexual health. This topic does not focus on prevention, (see http://www.cdc.gov/hiv/default.htm) or treatment issues (see http://www.thebody.com/). Together, the two websites cover a range of topics, from prevention techniques, resources and responses to commonly asked questions about HIV/AIDS and STIs. Although prevention and treatment issues are important, the goal of this topic is to help you understand how sexual health relates to your sexual behavior. To maintain and create sexual health, it is important to understand the thoughts you have about HIV, STIs and sexual behavior.

In the field of HIV/STI prevention, there is significant research into why people engage in unsafe sexual behavior. The research has generally suggested a number of themes relevant to sexual health including sexual compulsivity, mood, alcohol and drug use, and sexual functioning concerns.

In this approach, unsafe sexual behaviors are not the problem, but a symptom of something more. The relationship between sexual health and safer-sex behaviors can be multidirectional. For example, your mood can shape your sexual behavior, and your reaction to that behavior may set you up for the next round of your cycle. You might think, "I'm so ashamed of my behavior that my feelings of hopelessness and worthlessness have increased." The helpful part of this reality is that intervening in the process at any point is a start toward improving sexual health.

Working with others whose self-hatred, shame, guilt, depression and/or hopelessness contribute to their unsafe sexual behaviors has been one of my saddest experiences. I've heard too many times, "I wanted to kill myself by getting HIV." This is a classic example of why sexual health has so many components, and it highlights the difficulty many people have in moving toward sexual health. In these situations, sexual health requires addressing the underlying issues. Much of that material applies to safer-sex issues: "If I believe I'm worthless, and I can get affirmation through sex, I will do whatever my sexual partner wants in order to get them to stay with me, including breaking my personal guidelines for safer-sex."

While a depressed mood can contribute to high-risk behaviors, anxiety around HIV can cause some people to simply shut down their sexual expression. The anxiety leads to paralysis and fear. In some cases, the anxiety leads to sexual health concerns through ritual masturbation, sexual avoidance or use of sexually explicit material. The high level of anxiety in response to HIV can lead some people to use alcohol and drugs as a way to self-medicate and reduce the level of their anxiety. While under the influence, they might engage in unsafe sexual behavior that creates feelings of shame and guilt.

Assignment

- The last time you talked with your doctor about HIV/STIs was? The last time you were screened for HIV/STIs was? Your plans to speak with the doctor are:

- Review your unsafe sexual behavior. Reflect on the times you have engaged in unsafe sexual behaviors. Which reasons appear to be more relevant for you? Highlight at least 4–5 reasons for unsafe sexual behavior that are relevant to you.

- Examine the questions at the beginning of this section on page 64. For each question you scored a point, reflect on the underlying issues and identify plans to address the issues regarding why you scored the point.

- Examine your safer-sex behaviors through the lens of the values you want to shape your life. How consistent are these behaviors and values? If, for example, you value respect, how is self-respect impaired or damaged when you engage in unsafe sexual behaviors? How is respect for others diminished when you engage in unsafe sexual behaviors?

- Your personal safer-sex plans to address your unsafe sexual behavior are:

Chapter 4: Barriers to Sexual Health

While this book focuses on promoting sexual health, an honest self-assessment of possible barriers needs to occur. It is not possible to provide an exhaustive list of barriers to sexual health. What follows are the generally recognized barriers reflecting my understanding of the research and my clinical work. (Other clinicians might emphasize different aspects.) I group these barriers into compulsive behaviors, chemical use, mood disorders, and emotional, physical and/or sexual abuse. If any of these barriers are applicable, please seek the appropriate support and help.

Sexual Compulsivity: what is compulsive?

One person's compulsive behavior is another person's hobby. How do we really know what is healthy/unhealthy? The acting-out cycle is a framework to explain how people "act-out" their compulsive behaviors. Here is a brief review. Two workbooks focus on problematic sexual behavior: *Living a Life I Love* focuses on addressing sexual compulsivity in general and *Cybersex Unplugged* addresses internet compulsivity. Please see those resources for a deeper discussion and treatment approach.

When it comes to this particular field of treating problematic sexual behavior, coming up with a blanket definition and universal term is a challenge, mainly because there have been various terms that have been widely misused or overused. These most common terms include "sexual compulsivity," "sexual compulsion," and "love addiction." As a field, we have a range of accepted opinions. Generally, I prefer the term sexual compulsivity because I prefer to use a behavioral treatment approach. The following definition works in the majority of circumstances and provides a resource for individuals struggling with sexual problems. The definition of sexual compulsivity has two components: subjective and objective.

Subjective – Realization that a Problem Exists

On some level you recognize your sexual behavior is a problem. These behaviors often lead to feelings of guilt, shame, and self-recrimination. In psychology, we call this "ego-dystonic:" "I know I did something I didn't want to do.

Objective – External Notification of a Problem

You may not have realized there is a problem, but some form of external feedback has presented itself to bring the situation to light. This feedback can come in the form of a legal consequence (such as an arrest), a financial consequence (such as money spent on the Internet, or termination from a job) or damage to a relationship because of the violation of boundaries.

Sexual Avoidance

"How can I have a sex problem if I do not have sex?" Thoughts and feelings of shame, fear, and hopelessness can cause a person to avoid sexual contact. Sexual avoidance describes the state of depriving oneself of sex. One of the more difficult aspects of sexual avoidance is recognizing the problem. People easily know when they are not having sex, but they might not recognize that not having sex can mean they are out of control just as having sex can mean they are out of control. Sexual avoidance, or "sexual anorexia," is a less recognized and as a result less treated condition. Understanding the motivating factor underlying the lack of sex is what is important. The lack of sex is not important in itself. Often the underlying cause for sexual avoidance is similar to the cause for sexual compulsivity.

Chemical Dependency

Chemical dependency is a treatment issue in and of itself. If you struggle with chemical use I cannot overstate the importance of addressing this issue. The purpose of this section is to help you recognize any connections between your sexual behavior and chemical dependency by reviewing some of the indicators of chemical dependency, providing a screening tool, and then highlighting possible relationships between chemical dependency and sexual behavior. If appropriate, include chemical use in your timeline.

There is a distinction between chemical use, chemical abuse and chemical dependency. For example, you might drink alcohol and find there's nothing wrong with doing so. However, there might be times when you have engaged in unhealthy, risky or unwise behaviors while drinking. If this happens rarely, this might qualify for "chemical abuse." If you're level of use is higher, and you engage in a number of risky behaviors, or if the number of symptoms is higher, this might qualify as "chemical dependency."

It is important for you to identify your level of use, so that treatment options can be determined. The more severe the level of use, the more intensive the treatment option will need to be. A helpful tool is the classic alcohol-screening "CAGE" questionnaire derived from the following four questions:

- Have you ever felt you ought to *cut* down on your drinking?
- Have people *annoyed* you by criticizing your drinking?
- Have you ever felt bad or *guilty* about your drinking?
- Have you ever had a drink first thing in the morning to steady your nerves or get rid of a hangover (*eye-opener*)?

Give yourself one point for each "yes" answer. A total score of two or more is generally considered clinically significant and warrants further assessment.[6] A similar drug screen questionnaire can be found at the following link:

http://counsellingresource.com/quizzes/drug-abuse/index.html. Both screening tests are provided for your information. If your scores are higher, I strongly recommend you seek additional assessment and treatment if necessary.

The classic example is that someone may use alcohol, and then makes poor choices leading to sexual behavior. Another paradigm to consider is the alcohol use may be a response to negative thoughts that then leads to a series of sexual behaviors. Some individuals have VERY restrictive values or thoughts regarding sexuality. These thoughts lead to a behavior of "shutting down" or repressing sexuality. Once they use the chemicals, the ability to repress the thoughts and feelings decreases. In the first paradigm, chemical use appears to lead to sexual behavior. In the second paradigm, however, the restrictive sexual thoughts would be the primary problem with the chemical use being a secondary problem.

To highlight the need for an accurate assessment of the primary treatment issue, I point to clients I've worked with who have completed multiple chemical dependency treatments but who never dealt with issues of sexuality. With one client who could never maintain periods of chemical sobriety longer than a few months, it became clear that his sexual issues were more important to address than his chemical use issues.

Eating Disorders

With eating disorders, the person that often comes to mind is an adolescent female or young woman throwing up to reduce her weight because of bad body image. Although women account for the majority of eating disorders, the number of men with eating disorders is growing. Among gay men, the percentage is even higher.

Typically, eating disorders fall into three conditions: Anorexia Nervosa, Bulimia Nervosa and Eating Disorder, Not Otherwise Specified. Anorexia Nervosa is typically exhibited through the failure to eat or maintain proper nutrition. Bulimia Nervosa is typically exhibited through purging behaviors such as throwing up or laxative use. Most often, however, you will not find a person with an either/or diagnosis, hence the combined diagnosis of Eating Disorder, Not Otherwise Specified, which is sort of a catchall diagnosis.

Although it is difficult to accurately diagnose eating disorders, there are assessment tools. One researcher identified four questions that may be helpful. If you answer "yes" to three of the questions, she recommends you seek further assessment.[7]

1. Do you worry you have lost control over how much you eat?
2. Do you make yourself sick when you feel uncomfortably full?
3. Do you currently suffer with, or have you ever suffered in the past, from an eating disorder?
4. Do you ever eat in secret?

Part of addressing eating disorders will also require you to address the questions of body image discussed in the next chapter

Assignment

- Review your sex history and the timeline. Describe any relationship between your sexual behavior and chemical use, or other compulsive behaviors such as sexual compulsivity, online compulsivity, gambling or eating behaviors or body image?

- Do sexual behaviors trigger shame, which leads to chemical use or other compulsive behaviors?

Mental Health Factors

One of the largest barriers to sexual health is the presence of mental health factors. The four I focus on are: Attention Deficit Hyperactivity Disorder, Depression, Bi-Polar Disorder and Anxiety Disorders. The overlap between mood disorders and sexual health concerns is so common that the question is not, "Is there a mood disorder present?" but "*Which* mood disorder is present?" As with other areas discussed in the book, the connection between sexual behaviors and mental health concerns is probably bi-directional: people use sexual behavior to cope with a mental health concern; and sexual health issues contribute to increased mental health problems.

Mood disorder is the term used to describe a person's difficulty understanding, coping with, and managing a variety of feelings. Sometimes, people's feelings are out of control and they simply don't know what to do. Sexual behavior can be an attempt to cope with the feelings, or, vice-versa, the sexual behavior may trigger a series of feelings that appear out of control.

Understandably, some of my clients initially avoid a diagnosis of a mood disorder. The language and cultural response is often negative and judgmental. My request is that you be open to the possibility. Acknowledging a mood disorder might actually create hope because we have language to understand and strategies to treat the symptoms. You can search the Internet for basic screening instruments to help you further your self-discovery.

ADHD

Studies have reported an association between Internet compulsivity and attention deficit/hyperactivity disorder (ADHD). Most often, ADHD is first recognized in childhood or adolescence. Recently, adults are being diagnosed with ADHD more frequently. The diagnosis of adult ADHD is controversial, because the diagnosis of ADHD in adults is viewed by some as a "trendy" diagnosis rather than a true problem. Also, a diagnosis of adult ADHD is open to misuse, particularly when it provides an excuse for the behavior. E.g., "I go online because I have ADHD." To help you determine if you need follow-up, please review the following symptoms. If five or six of them describe you, please seek out and obtain the necessary support.

Symptoms of ADHD include:

- Does not give close attention to details.
- Makes careless mistakes in work, or other activities.
- Often has trouble keeping attention on tasks.
- Often does not seem to listen when spoken to directly.
- Often does not follow through on instructions.
- Fails to finish duties in the workplace.
- Often has trouble organizing activities.
- Doesn't want to do things that take a lot of mental effort.
- Often loses things.
- Is often easily distracted.
- Is often forgetful in daily activities.
- Often fidgets with hands or feet or squirms in seat when sitting still is expected.
- Often gets up from seat when remaining in seat is expected.
- Often feels very restless.
- Often has trouble doing leisure activities quietly.

- Is often "on the go" or often acts as if "driven by a motor."
- Often talks excessively.
- Often blurts out answers before questions have been finished.
- Often has trouble waiting one's turn.
- Often interrupts or intrudes on others (e.g., butts into conversations or games).

Depression

Without a doubt, a major issue related to sexual health is depression. In non-technical terms, statements such as "I'm sad" or "I don't have any energy" might be expressions of depression. Other behavioral indicators might be not eating or not getting out of bed. It is easy to see how sexual behavior can occur in response to feeling depressed, either through engaging in sexual behavior to feel good, or shutting down sexually. Sometimes the shame of sexual behavior may reflect a bigger issue of depression. The goal here is to review depression in such a way that you might recognize how depression and sexual health concerns are related.

One difficulty in recognizing the presence of depression is that sometimes depression may be part of a bigger issue. For example, the next issues I will cover are bipolar disorder, manic episodes and anxiety disorders. In each of these issues, depression may be a symptom of the other conditions. It may take some time for an accurate assessment that describes all of your symptoms. I've listed a number of symptoms below that are ranked according to seriousness of the symptoms. If three or more of these symptoms are present, I strongly recommend you seek additional help.

> **If you are experiencing suicidal thoughts, or feelings**, get immediate help at http://www.helpguide.org/mental/suicide_help.htm, call **1-800-273-TALK**, call **911** or visit your **local emergency room**. Suicidal thoughts are the most severe symptoms. Clinicians are trained to respond respectfully and immediately.

Symptoms of Depression (in descending order of severity):

- A suicide attempt.
- A specific plan for suicide.
- Recurrent suicidal ideation ("I want to die") without a specific plan.
- Recurrent thoughts of death (not just fear of dying).

- Depressed mood most of the day, nearly every day.
- People reporting to you that you look depressed.
- Feelings of irritability.
- Fatigue or loss of energy nearly every day.
- Feelings of worthlessness or excessive/inappropriate guilt.
- Loss of pleasure or interest in daily activities.
- Significant weight loss when not dieting (e.g., a change of more than 5% of body weight in a month).
- Decrease or increase in appetite nearly every day.
- Sleeping too much (can't get out of bed).
- Sleeping too little (can't fall asleep).
- Feelings of agitation; body is restless.
- No energy; body feels weary.
- Difficulty making decisions.
- Difficulty thinking or concentrating.

There are some issues that disqualify a mental-health diagnosis. Sometimes a more important/severe diagnosis takes priority. Or, if you've taken drugs or chemicals (e.g., alcohol), you might have a different diagnosis. In some cases, a medical condition might be a cause of some of the symptoms. Again, the key is to seek the advice of a professional if three or more of the above symptoms are present.

Bipolar Disorder/Manic Depression

Another mood disorder related to sexual health concerns is bipolar disorder. (The disorder is sometimes labeled "manic-depression.") As with anxiety and depression, bipolar disorder exists on a continuum of severity. Very few people experience the extreme form of the symptoms, officially labeled as "Bipolar I." My experience suggests that severe forms of bipolar disorder are difficult to manage and require a multidisciplinary approach including psychiatrists, therapists and a strong support network. The other forms of bipolar disorder are less-severe expressions and are probably more frequent and less recognized. Because they are less recognized, it is important to examine the descriptions and symptoms to see if one of the less-severe expressions might be present in relation to your sexual behavior. If symptoms are present, please check with a mental-health professional for further assessment and treatment.

Listed below are some symptoms of the manic episodes. If you experience three or more of these symptoms, please consult with a mental-health professional. If all the symptoms occur during the same time window (say, within a week), the "episode" may be labeled "manic." If the number of symptoms is fewer or the duration of the symptoms is shorter, the episode may be labeled "hypomanic." The intensity and number of symptoms often reflects the severity of the diagnosis.

- Increased energy, activity and restlessness.
- Excessively "high" euphoric mood.
- Extreme irritability.
- Racing thoughts and talking fast. Jumping from one idea to another.
- Distractibility; can't concentrate.
- Little sleep needed.
- Unrealistic beliefs in one's abilities and powers.
- Excessive self-esteem.
- Spending sprees.
- Increased sexual drive.
- Abuse of drugs, particularly methamphetamine, cocaine, alcohol and sleeping medications.
- Provocative, intrusive or aggressive behavior.
- Denial that anything is wrong.
- Overbearing behaviors that cross other people's boundaries.
- Dramatic increase in social or work-oriented activities.

Bipolar disorder usually reflects a swing from a manic to a depressive mood. Review the section on symptoms of depression. If you experience symptoms of both depression and bipolar disorder, a different treatment approach may be necessary. What makes bipolar disorder hard to assess is the difficulty recognizing a less-than-full-blown depressive episode or a less-than-full-blown manic episode. Individuals will often recognize signs of depression and obtain treatment for that condition, but are so grateful for the relief from the depression when in a manic or hypomanic stage that they don't see themselves as having further problems, such as bipolar disorder. Because of the emotional exhaustion of being in the depression stage, simply having energy is such a welcome relief for individuals with depression, that they do not seek further treatment.

Anxiety

Another important mood disorder to consider is anxiety and whether it has a role in your sexual behavior. Think about how anxiety is present and shapes your sexual behavior, or use of the Internet to avoid other sexual behavior. Anxiety, in the simplest sense, is a sense of fear or uneasiness. Some anxiety is helpful in that it motivates us. For instance, you might say, "I'm nervous that my boss will get upset if I don't complete the project by Friday, so I'm going to commit to completing it." In these cases, anxiety is a positive thing. In some situations, however, anxiety can be a serious problem for people. In extreme cases, anxiety disorders can be debilitating.

If anxiety becomes pronounced, it can express itself in various ways. For example, you may have trouble sleeping. You might find you dwell on a particular situation and find it difficult to concentrate on other things. Your appetite or eating behaviors might change. Alternatively, you might have a sense of vigilance or a feeling of impending disaster, as if "something bad is going to happen." In some cases, anxiety can mask other mental-health issues such as depression. Below are symptoms and types of anxiety. Ask yourself, "How do these symptoms show up in my life?" If you experience two or three symptoms, please seek professional help for additional consultation.

- Feelings of apprehension or dread.
- Trouble concentrating.
- Feeling tense and jumpy.
- Anticipating the worst.
- Irritability.
- Restlessness.

- Watching for signs of danger.
- Feeling like your mind's gone blank.
- Pounding heart.
- Sweating.
- Stomach upset or dizziness.
- Frequent urination or diarrhea.
- Shortness of breath.
- Tremors and twitches.
- Muscle tension.
- Headaches.
- Fatigue.
- Insomnia.

Treatment for Mood Disorders

Treatments for mental health issues vary. I encourage you to go online and search for strategies addressing the mental health issue relevant in your life. If you are working with a counselor, please ask about your counselor's level of expertise and comfort with a particular type of therapy. If you want to try something on the list below and your primary counselor can't provide the resources, it is your right to ask for a referral to a therapist who can. Here are a just a few possible treatment approaches:

Medication Management

The numbers and types of medications are constantly changing, so please consult with a trained professional. Many individuals are not interested in this treatment approach because of fear and stigma regarding medications, but at times the use of medication is appropriate. For example, let's say you've broken your foot. For a while, you'll need crutches for support as your foot heals. Think of medication as a similar support that can help you while you address the issues related to mood disorder. Also look at the example of diabetes treatment. Some people manage their diabetes through diet and exercise, and do not require medication. For some, however, long-term insulin use is required to stay healthy. Similarly, long-term use of medications may be needed for mental health. You and your doctor can work on the best fit and plan.

Talk Therapy

Talk therapy takes a range of approaches. The number and type of interventions are simply too many to list, but some of the better known therapies include:

- Cognitive-Behavioral Therapy (CBT).
- Dialectical and Behavioral Therapy (DBT) Skills.
- Supportive Talk Therapy.
- Eye Movement Desensitization and Reprocessing (EMDR) Therapy.
- Relationship Therapy.

Alternative Therapies

- Recreational Therapy Activities such as Challenge Courses.
- Eastern approaches such as Acupuncture, Yoga, and Massage.

Healthy Daily Activities[8]

One way to cope with mood disorders is to develop healthy habits that help balance the mood and create stability and balance in your life. Here are a few examples:

- Talk with someone. Ask trusted friends and acquaintances to spend time with you daily, preferably face to face.
- Wait until you are feeling better before attempting difficult tasks.
- Make a written schedule for yourself every day and stick to it.
- Get at least eight hours of sleep each night.
- Get out into the sun or into nature for at least 30 minutes a day.
- Make time for things that bring you joy.

Manage Your Diet

Managing your diet is another way to help with stabilizing your mood.

- Stop or reduce your consumption of products that contain caffeine, such as coffee, tea, cola and chocolate.

- Stop or reduce your consumption of products that contain nicotine (a stimulant).
- Review over-the-counter medicines or herbal remedies. Many contain chemicals that can affect mood.

Exercise/Relaxation

A holistic approach to treating mood disorders can facilitate balance, including:

- Exercise daily.
- Muscle tension is commonly experienced in the back of the neck and shoulders. One easy way to get rid of such tension is to tighten the neck and shoulders, holding for 5–10 seconds before releasing.
- Close your eyes, take a deep breath through the nose, exhale through your mouth and repeat a few times. When breathing in, let your stomach expand as much as possible. Concentrate on breathing slowly and calmly, thinking of your slow breathing as calming your entire body.

Meditation Activities

The activities in this section can help you focus your thoughts, as well as express feelings regarding factors associated with the mood disorder.

- Draw.
- Write in a Journal.
- Listen to relaxing music.
- Tell yourself "I am relaxed" as you carry out breathing exercises.
- Visualize a soothing image (e.g., lying on a warm beach).

Assignment

- In the sexual behavioral timeline (see page 31), you chart your life along the horizontal axis. The +5 to 0 range is to help you start thinking about the following topics. Look at the symptoms of ADHD, anxiety, depression and bipolar disorder. Which symptoms are present? Update your timeline by graphing these symptoms across your lifetime.

- As you review the material, reflect on how compulsive or addictive behaviors or feelings of depression, ADHD, anxiety and/or bipolar disorder symptoms relate to your sexual behavior.

- Could a mood disorder impair your sexual functioning?

- Might sexual behavior be attempts to reduce symptoms of the mood disorder?

- Might your sexual behaviors be a contributing factor to a mood disorder?

- Identify your plans to address any concerns raised in this topic.

Types and Impact of Abuse

It is important to review the relationship between abuse/neglect and your sexual time-line and sexual behavior. The topic of types and degrees of abuse and neglect are too complex for a complete discussion here, but the following is a brief review. The major types of abuse –physical, emotional, sexual – are categorized to help describe the abuse, but types of abuse may overlap. Please seek professional help if abuse or neglect is part of your history. Treatment approaches vary and are not reviewed here.

Physical Abuse

Physical abuse includes any behavior that causes or contributes to a physical injury to another person. The abuse can be direct or indirect. Direct abuse is when the perpetrator causes the physical contact. Indirect abuse is when a third object is involved. For example, if your neighbor hits you with her fist, she made *direct* contact with you. If she threw a lamp at you and missed, but to get out of the way you tripped, fell and bruised yourself, then she was an *indirect* cause of the injury. However, since she threw the lamp in the first place, she is ultimately a cause of the abuse.

Examples of physical abuse include the following:

- Getting hit.
- Getting hit with an object.
- Hair pulling.
- Being burned.
- Being cut.
- Someone stopping you from breathing for a short period of time.
- Administering a harmful substance
- Physical injury.
- Sexual Abuse

Sexual abuse can include a range of behaviors. These include extreme forms of abuse such as rape, molestation, forced prostitution or incest. Other forms of sexual abuse include exploitation, use of a power relationship (teacher/student, caretaker/child, therapist/client). Less extreme forms of abuse can include manipulation of others for sexual pleasure, voyeurism and exhibitionism. Sexual abuse also includes sexual harassment and verbal degradation. Sexual contact by an adult with a person under the legal age of consent is by statute a form of sexual assault and results in automatic criminal charges if revealed. Other examples of sexual abuse include the following:

- Sexual innuendoes or provocative statements.
- Engaging in sexual behavior in front of another person.
- Exposing one's genitals to another person without permission.
- Fondling or touching another's breast or genital area.
- An adult or older child engaging a child in sexual intercourse, masturbation, oral sex, or genital sex.
- Adult sexual contact, such as sexual intercourse, masturbation or oral-genital sex without permission or when permission is withdrawn.

Emotional Abuse

The third classic type of abuse is emotional abuse. This involves negative statements being directed toward you. Some incidents of emotional abuse might be one-time events, but often there is a pervasive pattern of negative statements. Examples of emotional abuse include the following:

- Name-calling.
- Put-downs.
- Failure to affirm.
- Shaming.
- Judgmentalism.
- Making threats.
- Yelling.

Overt and Covert Abuse

A lot of research and practice emphasizes addressing overt abuse, which is "abuse that is easily recognized." If you review the previous examples, it's easy to recognize whether something did or did not happen. There usually is a specific person, behavior, event, time and place when a person describes the abuse. In therapy, he/she will say, "My partner did. . . ." and then describe in great detail what happened.

Covert abuse is equally as damaging but is often hidden or covered and not recognized. We apply the label of covert abuse to any setting where there is an atmosphere of fear. Therefore, statements such "I can give you something to cry about" creates an atmosphere of impending physical abuse. Another example: "Don't make me get the belt." A third example is "Wait until your father gets home." These behaviors are covert physical abuse. The difficulty, however is that covert abuse is difficult to recognize. A person may sense something is wrong, but not have awareness of a specific problem. He or she may report being vigilant for no apparent reason. But the threat of abuse causes such an individual to shudder simply because of a look from a partner, friend, or parent. The threat or feelings of fear are the keys to recognizing covert abuse. Review each type of abuse. How might covert abuse be present in your life?

Abuse and Neglect

Abuse is typically an active behavior. (I "did" something, or something was "done" to me.) Just as damaging is neglect. Neglect is the failure to provide the necessary resources to another person. Emotional and physical neglect is often recognizable. Emotional neglect can be the failure to provide emotional support. Physical neglect can be the failure to provide appropriate nutrition, shelter or clothing. Sexual neglect could be the failure to provide adequate sexual education. Both covert abuse and neglect are very difficult to recognize. It is only after the fact and through the review of the indicators of abuse that a person can identify covert abuse and/or neglect.

Sexual Violence

Sexual violence is any type of sexual activity that you do not agree to. The amount of sexual violence in our society remains at epidemic proportions. Instances of sexual violence are notoriously underreported. Some scholars have suggested 3% of college women experience sexual assault in a given year.[9] Another article suggests 25% of girls and 16% of boys are abused before age 16.[10] Furthermore, professionals rarely recognize the concept of male-on-male rape as an issue and often do not provide treatment for victims.[11] Examples of sexual violence (usually referred to as sexual assault and abuse) include the following:

- Inappropriate touching (such as the grabbing of your breasts, butt or penis, or brushing up against you without your consent), whether it is intentional or *ostensibly* by accident.

- Vaginal, anal or oral penetration, or attempted penetration (with or without objects), without your consent.
- Being spied on (i.e., voyeurism).
- Having someone expose himself or herself to you without your consent.
- Sexual contact when consent is not present. (The concept of consent is covered in the topic, Sexual Behavior and Expression on page 120.)

Sexual violence can occur to anyone at any time. A relative or person known to the victim is the most common perpetrator of this kind of violence. When a partner, wife, husband or dating partner is the perpetrator, the abuse is defined as "domestic rape" or "date rape." The rise of date rape drugs exacerbates the problem and provides a barrier to seeking help. While sensationalized in the movies, stranger rape is less common, though it still occurs and is important to assess. If you are a victim of sexual violence, seek immediate help. Sometimes an individual does not seek immediate help for any number of reasons. It is never too late to seek help. This can include talking to a therapist, friend or religious advisor. The key is to remember that you are not alone, and that recovering from this experience is possible.

Indicators of Abuse

Below are typical symptoms that abused or neglected individuals experience. They are not always associated with abuse, but these are the early warning signs professionals look for. Review the indicators and compare them with your sexual history. If present, seek additional support.

Physical Indicators of Abuse

- Displays agitation or anger, uncontrollable behaviors, tantrums.
- Displays anxious behaviors (nail biting, teeth grinding, rocking, etc.).
- Often belittles self ("I'm bad, evil, etc.").
- Resists authority or desperately tries to please because they fear repercussions.
- Shows fear of a particular person or place.
- Thoughts involve themes of sexual acts, torture, bondage, humiliation and/or abuse.
- Hurts others sexually or physically.

- Acts aggressively around pets.
- A child mimicking adult sexual behavior (such as intercourse, French kissing, etc.).
- A child having age-inappropriate sexual knowledge.
- Increased chemical use.
- Increased sexual behavior.

Emotional Indicators of Abuse

- Individual has lots of new fears.
- Shows inappropriate emotions or no emotions at all.
- Fearful others hate them, are angry, want to hurt them, punish them or kill them.
- Fearful someone is "after them" or going to hurt them; wary of strangers.
- Has low self-esteem.
- Exhibits excessive guilt.
- Is unable to form friendships.
- Is self-destructive; intentionally inflicts harm on self.
- Appears to be "in a fog."
- Has excessive mood swings.
- Suicidal thoughts, statements or gestures

Personal Victimization History

The consequences of abuse vary, and can contribute to relationship, sexual and other problems. Sometimes a person's abuse history contributes to problematic sexual behaviors and chemical use. A common theme in sexual avoidance is a history of abuse. Due to an experience of abuse, a person may have difficulty recognizing and expressing feelings and empathizing with others. Often, people may not label the events as abuse because they don't recognize that they aren't at fault. They say they liked or respected the perpetrator or they could not believe the person would harm them. Sometimes a person thinks the abuse is a normal part of life. Victims have sometimes reported feelings of confusion because they liked the attention or they physically responded to the sexual touch.

Review the above indicators of abuse. Consider if any indicators are present. Might there be a particular event or source of the indicators? To recover from abuse, work with a therapist trained to address these issues.

Post Traumatic Stress Disorder

Given the powerful consequences of trauma, the impact on a person's sexual health cannot be underestimated. The severity of PTSD requires support and the intervention of mental health professionals. As you move through the treatment process, please speak with a clinician who can support you. The general concepts of PTSD are that you experienced a traumatic event, have flashbacks about the event and the reaction to the experience negatively affects your functioning. If something like this has occurred in your life, please consult with an expert.

Recovery from Abuse

If you are in immediate danger, you need a safe place. There are treatment programs, and/or shelters available. Look for Domestic Abuse or Sexual Violence programs in your local area. I encourage you to find help. My experience is that this can be a significant process for many individuals.

Once stable, tell your story. And then tell your story again and again. Group support/therapy is helpful. The decrease in shame, fear and isolation that occurs through group therapy can be powerful. Understanding that "I'm not alone" and "Someone understands" is a powerful source of hope. I often have clients complete an "abuse history" describing the life history of abuse. For some people this is too difficult. I acknowledge that healing is a long process. Sharing your story once is only the start. If you need to start slowly, simply listing events is the place to start. In such instances, I adapt the assignment by asking, "Describe 4 (or whatever number) events of abuse in your life." Sometimes, simply acknowledging, "I've been abused" is the first step.

Once you know your history, understand the things that trigger flashbacks and struggles in your current daily functioning. You'll need to develop plans to address the triggers. As you move forward, ask yourself what you want your life to look like.

This is the hardest place to get to in therapy. The level of fear and lack of hope will need to be resolved prior to this place.

Journaling has two benefits. It is part of the therapy process, but it also helps to remind you of your progress. When you are frustrated, it is helpful to look back and recognize where you've been, what you've come through, and where you're going. Some individuals "beat themselves up" because they can't talk to everyone at a party because they are uncomfortable. A journal can highlight the amazing progress signified by simply getting to an event. Journaling doesn't have to mean writing. With new technologies, journaling can include video recordings, art or other forms of expression.

Assignment

- For stable (i.e., not experiencing suicidal thoughts or showing major symptoms of post-traumatic stress disorder) individuals, I suggest they work on an abuse history. Include details such as your age, who, what, when, where and your reaction at the time. Update your timeline as appropriate. Also include your reaction today. Reflect on how the abuse affected you, and identify how it has influenced your sexual behavior. In writing your abuse history, include:

  - Physical, sexual, emotional abuse.
  - Overt and covert abuse.
  - Experiences with both abuse and neglect.
  - Experiences of sexual violence

- Have you experienced sexual violence? What changes in your life occurred as a result? What help have you received? What help would you have liked to receive? What help do you need?

- Have you experienced any major life threatening events? Review your sexual history. Highlight any events you continually re-experience? This might include nightmares, flashbacks, daydreams or startling thoughts.

- Has there been a change in your level of comfort with sexual behavior? Are there behaviors you now avoid?

- Has there been a change in your level of comfort with touch?

- Has there been a change in your level of emotional expression?

- Are there individuals who trigger an emotional response simply at the sight of them? Why do they trigger this response?

- As appropriate, what are your plans to address these issues?

Use of the Internet and Other Technology

The growing use of the Internet and impact on sexuality resulted in a separate volume addressing the unique characteristics of Internet Sexual Compulsivity. If this is a major problem, *Cybersex Unplugged* might be a better workbook for you. An overview is provided here. In the years since its wide integration into all aspects of our life, the Internet has provided easy access for all types of sexual content. For some people this is not a problem, but for others this access has only increased the amount of their unhealthy behavior. When you look at your Internet use, consider the following questions:

Assignment

- Review the questions on Internet Related Sexual Behaviors on page 27. What behaviors did you identify?

- What devices have you used to access explicit material (phone, computer, etc.)?

- How have you attempted to restrict or otherwise cut back your amount of Internet use? Were you successful?

- How are you using the Internet for sexual behaviors, which, if discovered, would create serious consequences (e.g., relationship issues, discipline at work)?

- How has the Internet set up other problematic behaviors (e.g., Internet to sex to drug use)?

- What are your plans to address the Internet as a treatment issue? Discuss your plan with your support network.

Behavioral Analysis

As I mentioned, there is no way to identify all possible barriers to sexual health, but a helpful tool in identifying such barriers is the completion of a behavioral analysis. This is a step-by-step examination of what happens in an unhealthy experience. The goal is to help you identify relevant issues, so you should examine all details, no matter how small you think they are.

I often challenge my clients to tell me how to drive a car. As they do, I playfully trip them up by asking questions about this or that. What they come to realize is that driving a car is a remarkably complex task that calls for multiple thought processes requiring you to pay attention to details. In psychology, this term is called "automaticity," the ability to complete complex behaviors without active cognitive thinking. It's like a habit. The behavioral analysis is a way to slow down and uncover the contributing factors underlying the behavior.

In the process of completing the analysis, you will identify a number of places to intervene to help improve your sexual life. The example below highlights multiple ways you may have failed to cope with the thoughts, feelings or related high-risk circumstances throughout a given time period. The key, then, is to identify ways you can interrupt any and all of the various unhealthy aspects of sexual health.

Instructions

To complete the analysis, it may be helpful to work backwards. Start with the incident. Answer the question "What happened?" Then ask, "What happened right before that?" and so on. Stay focused on what happened while you work backward. Don't give up to early, but you can always add more if you remember. It's like tracing the last domino's fall back to the first domino. Once you have a good start at what happened, complete the other columns by adding the corresponding thoughts, triggers and circumstances. Try to fill each column, but if you can't you can always come back to it. At the end of the process, summarize the behavioral analysis. Every item in the analysis becomes a place to develop a plan to help you move forward.

What Happened	What Were You Thinking	What Where you Feeling	Describe the Scene
I wake up tired.	I did it again.	Shame. Hopelessness.	Isolation. Avoid my support network.
I bring someone home. I don't use condom.	He/she is attractive. Sex will be great.	Excited, happy, numb, distracted.	Unsafe Sex. Not establishing boundaries.
I look around while at the bar.	Maybe I can connect with someone.	Lonely, excited	Cruising.
I head over to the bar after work.	Maybe I can meet some of my friends.	Lonely, tired, sad.	Bar setting.
I shut down.	Can't talk to anyone. I'm alone.	Sad, depressed, lonely, tired.	Isolation.
Boss mad at me.	I can't do anything right. She found out	Fear, sadness, shame, guilt.	Seeing someone angry.
I hide the mistake.	Maybe they know.	Fearful again.	Lying.
I drink at lunch.	At least I won't feel anything for a while.	Relaxed, calm.	Drinking.
Boss angry (and not even at me).	Better be careful or she'll turn on me. I'd better not screw up.	Worried/fearful that someone is angry.	Someone is angry
Went to work		Tired.	
Woke up tired; Didn't sleep well.	Frustrated that I didn't sleeping well.	Tired.	Not Sleeping Well.
Summary of the analysis	**Catastrophizing. Minimizing. I can't make a mistake. I'm in trouble. I can't tell anyone. I'm going to get fired. I'm alone.**	**Lonely. Tired. Worried. Anxious. Fearful. Sad. Depressed. Lonely. Shame. Hopelessness. Excited.**	**Not sleeping well. Making a mistake. Isolation. Being in a bar. Drinking. Cruising. Unsafe Sex.**

Chapter 5: Internal Factors of Sexual Health

This section is designed to focus on aspects of sexual health that are internal factors. This is simply a way to group the topics of Body Image, Masturbation, Fantasy and Sexually Explicit Material. In these sections, you are encouraged to look at your beliefs, values, and sexual behaviors related to these topics.

Body Image

A major component of sexual health is body image. Sexual health involves challenging the stereotypical and cultural images of beauty and encouraging self-acceptance. In order to do this you have to develop a realistic and positive body image. The necessary work in moving toward sexual health suggests this is a major issue for many people. Body image is the foundation for so many parts of our perceptions, internal messages, external messages and feelings that its impact is difficult to address.

Respond YES or NO to the following statements:

1. In general, I like how my body looks.
2. I like the look of my genitals.
3. I feel I am too thin.
4. I like how my breasts/chest looks.
5. I am uncomfortable with several parts of my body.
6. It is important for me to make my body look good.
7. I have had cosmetic surgery to change my looks.
8. Overall, I feel my body is attractive.
9. FOR MEN: I like the size of my penis.
    FOR WOMEN: I like the size of my breasts.
10. I want to look more masculine.
11. I want to look more feminine.

Score 1 point for each "no" answer to statements 1–4 and 6–9. Score 1 point for each "yes" answer to statements 5, 10–11. The higher the score, the bigger is the concern with body image issues.

What is considered beautiful changes culturally across time. The key to addressing body image is to acknowledge the role of culture (see page 36) and that beauty is based entirely on thought (review the Power of Thought on page 33). Clients who struggle with sexually explicit media will often place unrealistic expectations on themselves and their partners. The role of sexually explicit material, including the Internet's ability to flash images of the perfect body, raises concerns because of the impact it has in shaping people's view of their bodies. I hear significant numbers of stories about individuals struggling with accepting their own body image, as well as the body image of their partner. Intrinsic in the cultural messages we receive is the idea that an attractive body is limited to a youthful body. Other negative thoughts we may have about ourselves as a result of cultural messages include, "My penis is too small," and "My breasts aren't ok." Without a doubt, mainstream American culture worships the perfect body and sets unrealistic expectations for both men and women. In our culture, the objectification of women has been occurring for a while. Recent developments have shown the objectification of men as well. Given the cultural emphasis on unrealistic body images, the negative messages both genders face are tremendous.

Researchers examine factors contributing to body image struggles. Research suggests that a person's self-image is linked to the partner's response. Negative reactions from partners led to increased struggles with body image. As one could guess, individuals who struggle with body image issues have a better response to treatment progress when they have the support of a primary romantic partner. Individuals who receive such support have less stress and anxiety.

There are three implications that are important. First, for individuals who struggle with body image issues, the key is to gain support from the primary partner. Second, if the partner isn't supportive, it is important to address the negative impact of the partner's behavior. Hearing "You're fat" isn't going to help. Third, partners are also pummeled by the same cultural messages. Partners may need training and education as well as feedback regarding providing the necessary support.

Much of this appears to be common sense. Explicit positive and negative messages about a person's body can easily be recognized for what they are. The difficulty, however, lies is recognizing implicit, hidden, or subtle positive or negative messages. For individuals struggling with sexual health concerns, assessing the messages you see from your sexual behavior is important.

While a lot of people struggle with obtaining the ideal body, as dictated by their culture, a mental health diagnosis reflects significant body image issues. Body Dysmorphic Disorder is characterized by constantly comparing your appearance with that of others, possibly refusing to let your picture be taken, excessive checking of a certain body part that you think is flawed (e.g., your nose or belly), feeling anxious and self-conscious around other people, calling yourself names or having plastic surgery and then feeling dissatisfaction with the results of plastic surgery. If this is an issue, please work with a mental health professional.

Developing a Healthy Body Image

Following are some ideas that can help you work toward a positive body image:[12]

- Listen to your body. Eat when you are hungry.
- Be realistic about the size you are likely to be based on your genetic and environmental history.
- Exercise regularly in an enjoyable way, regardless of your size.
- Expect normal weekly and monthly changes in weight and shape.
- Work toward self-acceptance and self-forgiveness — be gentle with yourself.
- Ask for support and encouragement from friends and family when life is stressful.
- Decide how you wish to spend your energy — pursuing the "perfect body" or enjoying family, friends, school and, most importantly, life?

Assignment

- Read the discussion on Sexually Explicit Material (see page 97). How do images in sexually explicit media shape your image of the human body? How do they shape how you see your body?

- How do images of sexually explicit media shape how you see your partner's body?

- Examine your sexual history. How have messages regarding body image affected your sexual behavior?

- How have these messages led to avoidant behaviors?

- List 25 negative thoughts you have about your body or hear from your culture(s). The goal is to help you become aware of the amount of negative self-talk.

- List a positive thought for each negative thought you have about your body or hear from your culture(s).

- Identify two plans you will do to create a healthy body image?

What would your genitals say?

Within the concept of body image is genital image. Sexual health includes a healthy acceptance of your genitals. When we talk about genitals, I include a broad understanding including not only the vagina/penis area (pelvic), but also the anus and buttocks, and (while not technically included but still helpful) breast/chests/nipples. People have an aversion to looking at, or otherwise being aware of their own genitalia. Some of the most often mentioned reasons for the aversion to genitals include the following.

• Because of abuse, some individuals struggle with being a sexual being. The topic of genitals is reduced to sex, and something to be avoided.

• Masturbation is such a taboo topic that anything associated with it becomes taboo.

• Other individuals struggle with porn images either in real time or from the Internet. The comparison to these bodies and genital images impacts are view of breasts, stomachs, chests, penises, and buttocks. The thought is usually, "I don't look like that so I will be rejected."

A number of exercises have developed to increase acceptance of genitals. In the movie "Fried Green Tomatoes" the character played by Kathy Bates is encouraged to use a mirror to examine her vagina in the goal of accepting her femininity. While we may laugh, the exercise has at its core the concept of self-acceptance and self-knowledge, including your genitals. To improve your genital image, get to know them better! This can include taking pictures, touching them in a self-discovery way, identifying what parts you find pleasurable. Pay attention to more than just the pelvic area but include your buttocks, anus, and breast/chest area. With a partner, have them touch your genitals to help you discover what you like, including the types of touch.

Assignment

As you move forward in sexual health, especially over the next few chapters pay attention to your beliefs and feelings of your genitals. Consider the following questions.

- What thoughts and feelings do I have about my genitals?

- What barriers do I have toward healthy acceptance of my genitals?

- What do I see as a healthy genital image?

- What are two plans I will implement to improve my genital image?

Masturbation

American culture has a significant amount of negative beliefs regarding masturbation. An article that presents the basics and history of masturbation is at Wikipedia (http://en.wikipedia.org/wiki/Masturbation). The focus of this section is to examine the role of masturbation in your sexual life. It is also important to examine your thoughts and the historical messages you have received about masturbation and to examine how these thoughts have helped or hindered your sexual health.

Respond YES or NO to the following statements:

1. I enjoy masturbating.
2. Masturbation is a good way to affirm my sexuality.
3. Masturbation is a good way to help me feel better about myself.

4.   I believe masturbation is sinful.

5.   Masturbation is a healthy way to have sex when I'm horny.

6.   Masturbation is a good way to get to know what a sexual partner likes.

7.   Masturbation with my sexual partner(s) is a healthy expression of being close to each another.

8.   Masturbation is very safe sex.

9.   Masturbation is a healthy way to learn about my sexual desires.

10.   Masturbation is a positive source of comfort and pleasure.

11.   Masturbation is a form of healthy sexual expression.

12.   Masturbation can be helpful in overcoming sexual dysfunction.

13.   I masturbate to explore my body.

14.   I masturbate too much.

15.   I feel guilty when I masturbate.

16.   Masturbation is a good way to reduce stress.

17.   Masturbation is a good form of birth control.

Score 1 point for each "yes" response to statements 1–3, 5–13 and 16–17. Score 1 point for each "no" response to statements 4, 14, 15. The higher your score, the more comfortable you are with masturbation.

The questions above are a good place to start in assessing your views about masturbation. Review each question again, giving attention to your reaction. Review your sex history and the questions about masturbation. As you examine the responses, pay attention to your past and current thoughts and feelings about masturbation. For some people, masturbation is a form of harm reduction. By masturbating, they know they will reduce the risk of other sexual health problems.

Often partners will have different opinions in addressing masturbation. Some say that masturbation is a healthy outlet within a relationship and that it should be incorporated into the relationship with their partner. Masturbation can be a way to discover what you like sexually, as well as what parts of your body are most arousing or sensitive. In this example, masturbation can lead to a heightened awareness of self that can be shared with your partner. In other opinions, masturbation is a form of settling when the primary partner is unavailable. One example is a guideline within a relationship where you ask the partner if he/she is available for sex. If the partner says, "no," then masturbation is allowed. Still other approaches view masturbation as a sin.

The key to the following questions is to clarify your opinions, beliefs and values about masturbation. Think about the role of masturbation in your definition of sexual health.

Assignment

- Review the discussion on Culture (see page 36). Identify 2 messages about masturbation from each culture you belong to.

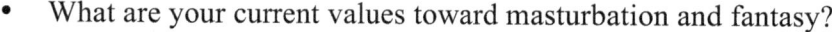

- What are your current values toward masturbation and fantasy?

- Describe the content and format of sexually explicit material you've used while masturbating. Explain if this is healthy or unhealthy.

- Under what circumstances is masturbation healthy for you?

- Under what circumstances is masturbation unhealthy for you?

- What are your current appropriate masturbation behaviors? (Where, when, how often?)

- What are your guidelines about disclosing masturbation behaviors to your partner?

- What is my partner's reaction to these guidelines?

Fantasy

Respond YES or NO to the following statements:

1. If I fantasize about sex, I will become obsessed about sexual thoughts.
2. It is difficult for me to share my sexual fantasies with my sexual partner(s).
3. Sharing a sexual fantasy with my sexual partner(s) enriches my sex life.
4. Sexual fantasy helps me learn about what I like and don't like sexually.
5. Sharing a sexual fantasy is a good way to get to know what a sexual partner likes.
6. I enjoy fantasizing about sex.
7. I feel guilty when I fantasize about sex.
8. I enjoy hearing about my sexual partner's sexual fantasies.
9. Sexual fantasy helps me express my sexual desires.
10. Sexual fantasy is a safe outlet for sexual behaviors I choose not to act on.

Score 1 point for each "yes" response for statements 3–7 and 9–10. Score 1 point for each "no" response for statements 1, 2 and 8. The higher your score, the more comfortable you are with sexual fantasies.

The idea of sexual fantasies has many negative societal biases and messages that need to be confronted. In moving toward sexual health, it is important to clarify misperceptions that exist about fantasies. Having fantasies does not mean you are "oversexed," even if you fantasize or think about sex often.

Generally speaking, fantasies are normal aspects of our sexuality. Everybody has fantasies and daydreams. In fact, if you engage in online behaviors, _**all**_ of your Internet behavior is based on fantasy! Seriously, I cannot stress enough that all of you online behavior is related to fantasy. Given the conduit, all of the chat, pictures, and experiences exist in a realm where the mind has to fill in the blanks to make the experience feel real. Often online sexual behaviors lead to such intense fantasies that the fantasies take on an obsessive quality leading to the exclusion of real face-to-face intimacy.

Fantasies themselves are neutral. They are normal and healthy. At the same time, it is important to emphasize that some fantasies are risky or unhealthy. For some, there is such an imbalance, significant therapy needs to focus on addressing the fantasy content. The content, frequency, intensity and focus of the fantasy may raise issues you need to address. Fantasies can be helpful in understanding your sexuality. By examining your fantasies you can get a sense of what you find arousing. You can understand your needs and share them with your partner and support network. Sometimes a person can channel his or her energy into sexual fantasies to allow a healthy release. Sharing fantasies is difficult for some people, yet the process of sharing your fantasies can create positive intimacy with your partner.

Sexual fantasies are thoughts and feelings about sexual behaviors and ideas we find sexually arousing. Sexual fantasies may represent what turns us on. Sexual fantasies are also a form of self-stimulation. Simply having a fantasy does not mean we have to act on that fantasy. Fantasies exist only in thoughts; they are not in themselves real. This also means that a fantasy about a negative traumatic event is also not real.

I distinguish between a sexualization and a sexual fantasy by using a "three-second rule." The three-second rule refers to the amount of time you think about a person. What transforms a sexualization into a sexual fantasy is the thought or fixation on a particular person, image or object. If the thought is less than three seconds, it is a sexualization. If it is longer than 3 seconds, it is a fantasy. I came up with the three-second rule in response to others asking for a helpful guideline on when the process switches from a sexualization to a fantasy. I base this rule on clinical experience and not necessarily on any hard and fast research. Nor does it have to be three seconds: it could be two or four seconds.

Sexualizations are normal, they happen outside our realm of control and they're part of our sexual drive. Sexualizations simply happen. Throughout the day, many sexualizations occur. A sexualization is recognition that someone is attractive to you. Often sexualizations can occur outside one's primary sexual partner template. A straight man can recognize a handsome guy, just as a gay man can recognize a beautiful woman. In these situations, there is simply recognition of the sexuality and sensuality of another person. It is our response to the sexualization that raises issues for further treatment.

If a person uses sexual fantasies to avoid or escape from reality, or the fantasies are one's only form of sexual expression, then we have some concern. Some people use fantasies as a form of escape from unpleasant thoughts and feelings. The key is for you to figure out which fantasies are healthy and which are unhealthy.

Occasionally, thoughts of inappropriate or unhealthy behaviors may occur as themes in your fantasies. This is an important issue for individuals with a pattern of sexually offending behavior. It is also true for people in chemical dependency recovery when sexual fantasies include drug use. How you respond to the unhealthy fantasies is a key step toward sexual health. You can redirect and change the fantasy through changing the "plot" of the fantasy. If you find that you cannot do this, it is important that you stop the fantasy and avoid actively encouraging the unhealthy fantasy. Changing your environment and talking with your network can help you avoid these unhealthy fantasies. If you recognize that unhealthy fantasies are increasing in frequency, intensity or content, let your support system know you're having unhealthy or risky fantasies can be a part of creating sexual health

In our fantasies, we can create and clarify our values regarding sexuality and our relationship with others. Jack Morin identifies the concept of "core erotic thought," which he uses to demonstrate how our thoughts shape our sexual fantasies. Examining our most powerful fantasies gives us insight into how we see our basic selves. In his book, *Erotic Mind*, Morin discusses how fantasies changed in light of the therapeutic process. Specifically, he describes how negative and damaging fantasies slowly decrease as clients address underlying issues. As the clients move toward health, Morin suggests that the fantasies changed as a result of the therapeutic work. The goal for this section is to emphasize not only the importance of acknowledging the fantasies, but also the importance of studying them in order to gain insight into our underlying patterns of thinking and move toward sexual health. Consider the following possibilities: Fantasies may be a form of online harm–reduction. Fantasies may be a form of alternative sexual expression. Or, fantasies may be a form of avoidance. You need to clarify the role of fantasy in your life.

Assignment

Identify three highly arousing fantasies you've had recently. I encourage you to write 2-3 pages per fantasy with as much detail as possible. Complete a behavioral analysis on the fantasy (see page 91). Consider the following questions:

- What is the content of the fantasy? Explain the five "Ws": who, what, when, why, where.

- If this fantasy were to become a reality what would you think and feel as a result?

Sexually Explicit Material

One of the more controversial issues in the field of sexual health is the role and use of sexually explicit material (I describe this below). Notice the language: I use the phrase "sexual explicit material" to describe any content used in a sexual manner instead of using the problematic term "pornography." (Pornography is often assumed to be limited to nude magazines or nude videos.) I use this approach for two reasons. One reason for the change in language is to step beyond the controversy of the language, and second highlight the need to assess adequately the use of ANY material a person sees as sexually explicit or might use in a sexually stimulating way.

The shear number of explicit images of all kinds is phenomenal. Sexually explicit material includes sex images, but it also includes benign advertisements such as images from catalogs, storefronts or billboards. The number of individuals who report they looked at bra ads while growing up demonstrates how material can be sexually explicit without being pornographic. Some find the models in Victoria's Secret and Abercrombie & Fitch advertising sexually arousing. Or, likewise, Men's Health magazine or the Sports Illustrated Swimsuit Issue. Although these images are not nude, people do use them for sexual purposes, including masturbation and fantasy.

Experts have differing opinions on the use of sexually explicit material. Some clinicians believe any and all sexually explicit material is unhealthy because it exploits others and can be misused. Some religious traditions believe that looking at sexually explicit material is tantamount to infidelity and therefore is a sin (equivalent to "coveting your neighbor's wife"). Other clinicians have a neutral reaction to the use of sexually explicit material and focus on the surrounding context. Still other clinicians use sexually explicit material to educate couples and to help them address sexual functioning issues and facilitate the sharing of sexual thoughts with a partner. For the sake of this exercise, I define "sexually explicit" as any material you use for sexual arousal or which you sexualize (see the section on Fantasy on page 101).

The role of sexually explicit material in your life plays a part in your sexual health. My approach is to help you identify your current use of sexually explicit material, review your values regarding the material and focus on the role of the material in your sexual health. Taking on the values that (you think) others hold or what you think they want you to hold only sets you up for failure. Frequently, I have worked with clients who present as having an Internet problem, because their partner objects to sexually explicit material. Usually this means the work focuses on the relationship concerns versus the online behavior.

Assignment

Review your sex history and timeline; highlight the types and amount of sexually explicit material you've used. As you increase your awareness of the type and amount of material, also focus on what you find arousing or attractive. As mentioned, the content can range from pictures, videos, online materials, stories, advertising material and even art. As a starting point in your personal assessment, start with an extremely conservative definition of sexually explicit material. Note any medium with content you sexualize. Focus on how much material you explicitly seek out versus material simply present in your environment. The key is to help you highlight the degree to which sexual content is present in your life. It might be important to include this in your timeline.

- What sexually explicit material have you used?

- Highlight any corresponding thoughts, feelings, fantasies or memories that come to mind when you view this material. What themes are present?

- What are my current values toward sexually explicit material?

- What sexually explicit material is acceptable to use? Why?

- What sexually explicit material is not acceptable to use? Why?

- What are my guidelines about disclosing my use of sexually explicit material to my partner? Have I reviewed these guidelines with my partner? Does he/she agree with these values? If there is disagreement, what is my plan to address the disagreement?

Chapter 6: Positive Sexuality

Positive Sexuality

In this section, the focus of the conversation is to help you think about what you want. Here I want to you focus on what is right in your life versus what is wrong. The goal is to help you get your sexual needs met in a healthy way.

To understand positive sexuality, first we must understand sexuality in a brand new way – as a normal, vital, and positive aspect of your life. Too many people suffer pain when they think about sexuality. Give yourself permission to be a sexual being. Rather than repressed, hidden or shamed, positive sexuality celebrates your sexual energy and being. Yes, this includes sexual behavior, but it includes much more.

The key to this section is discovery. As I referenced in the section of discernment (see page 9) this is your chance to engage in play. Sex is adult play, so check out what you like or don't like. Enjoy the positive experiences, and let go of the unpleasant experiences. Pay attention to what energizes you, makes you feel alive, leaves you light-hearted, reflects integrity in your life, and can be shared with your support network.

Your task in this section is to challenge most, if not all of the messages you have heard about sexuality. This doesn't mean you have to discard your beliefs. Instead, understand both the letter and spirit of the messages. Sexual health is a journey. Today's thoughts are for today. What you like today is for today. What you want is for today. You have the privilege of addressing tomorrow's likes and wants tomorrow.

Balance is important in the journey. You can change your mind on this journey. I place good/bad sexual experiences on a different continuum than the continuum of healthy/unhealthy. You can have a sexual encounter that feels good but is unhealthy (think meth/sex), and a bad experience that is healthy (think too tired to function, but emotional intimacy). My hope is that you have great experiences along the way. Sometimes, the only way we know what is sweet is because we can compare it to what is sour. Enjoy your journey in sexual health!

Why Have Sex?

Sexuality is a powerful force in our life. As with any part of our life, there can be many reasons to engage in a particular behavior. This is essentially answering the question, "Why have sex?" While the reasons for having sex are often oversimplified, it is important for you to uncover some of the reasons you might engage in sexual behavior. In some circumstances, the reasons for having sex may highlight clinical issues that you need to address. This is a much more difficult task than you may think. To put this in perspective, a recent journal article identified 237 reasons a person has sex and identified four groups of reasons why people have sex, as follows:[13]

Physical reasons for sex:

- Stress Reduction. "I am at work, and this gives me a distraction."
- Pleasure. "Sex is fun." "Having an orgasm is fun."
- Physical Desirability. "I want that person." "That person wants me."
- Experience Seeking. "I'm bored and don't have anything to do." "I can do something online that I wouldn't do in person."

Goal attainment for sex:
- Resources. "I will get money/drugs."
- Social Status. "My reputation will get better." "No body will know."
- Revenge. "I will make that other person mad."
- Utilitarian. "I will get a raise/promotion."

Emotional reasons for sexual behavior:
- Love and Commitment. "I love you." "I'm scared of my partner."
- Expression of Feelings. "I'm sorry." "I'm mad at my partner"

Insecurity reasons for sex:
- Self-Esteem Boost. "Someone wants me, I feel better."
- Duty/Pressure. "My partner won't do what I want."
- Mate Guarding. "I can't have sex with my partner, so I'll go online instead."

Notice that what is a payoff depends on the person. While some payoffs may appear similar across individuals, each person has their own unique goals. Review your sexual timeline and history. Examine which reasons for sexual behavior may be relevant. As you reflect on the reasons, examine your thoughts and assumptions. If, for example, a reason for sexual behavior is to increase self-esteem, examine the thoughts and feelings associated with the low esteem.

Assignment

- Review your sexual timeline for any possible payoffs listed above.

- What are your initial plans to help you get these payoffs in healthy ways?

Assertive Communication

In moving toward sexual health, it is important to develop assertive communication skills while avoiding passive, aggressive and passive/aggressive communication patterns. This is relevant not only to expressing thoughts and feelings but also relevant to expressing yourself sexually. It is important to communicate with your partners your sexual likes and needs. At first, this style of communication may feel artificial. I encourage you to view it as a template and helpful tool. There are many formulas that can be helpful in learning assertive communication. I like the following template:

1. I am committed to__(a few words on why you are doing this)___.

2. I think/I feel____(state your thought or feeling).

3. Because____(explain what triggered the thought or feeling).

4. I need/want/would like___(express the request).

5.   I commit to __(identify how you will help this person be successful)__ .

Each statement has its own purpose for developing a stronger relationship and eventually helping you get your needs met.

In statement #1, think about the times when you've received helpful feedback. Typically you trusted that or knew these people were on your side. Reminding your listener of your goal helps them understand that the assertive communication is focused on growth: "In terms of a relationship, I'm committed to a loving relationship." Statement #2 is about being self-aware, about asking "What's going on inside?" It may be a thought, feeling or memory triggered by the current moment. Your ability to answer the question is improved by the mindfulness exercises (see page 34). Statement #3 should be a simple explanation of the moment, "short and sweet" and explicitly connected to the moment. If it takes more than one breath to say it, then it's too long. Statement #4 is a request, and the key is to be clear, specific and measurable. Again, if it takes more than one breath, then it is too long. Bear in mind distinctions among 'needs', 'wants' and 'likes'. Often, language confuses the importance of something. Someone says, "I *need* a cell phone," but in reality, they merely *want* or *would like* a cell phone. A need is a basic requirement for existence: "I need food," or "I need respect" or "I need you to stop touching me." Finally, statement #5 declares how you will help the other person be successful, something you will do to support the goal. It can include such statements as, "I will tell you when I want to be touched," or, "I will tell you what I like instead of making you guess." Helping the person be successful reconnects you to Statement #1. The template builds the relationship.

There are a few pitfalls to avoid. First, it is important to avoid the passive approach toward communication. A classic danger is the phrase "Would you like to ...?" instead of "I would like . . ." or "I expect ..." Other unhelpful forms of communication are "We" statements. Use "I" statements instead. Equally important is to avoid aggressive communication, including the manner of the communication (i.e., loud, yelling) or language such as " You" statements which are often more aggressive. "You should . . ." is better replaced with "I want" or "I need."

Assertively expressing your requests is a significant component of sexual health. Setting boundaries and setting limits can have major impacts on relationships. Assertiveness is important in expressing feelings and sexual desires. I have provided only a brief introduction to the concept. If the topic is relevant to you, or if you have significant struggles with assertive communication, please follow up with your support network.

Assignment

- Examine your sexual history. How is the lack of assertiveness related to your behaviors?

- Identify times when you have engaged in passive, aggressive or passive/aggressive behaviors. How could you change these encounters into assertive communication?

- What is the role of thoughts and feelings in your ability to be assertive? Could shame (see page 44) be present? If you feel shame, you might be hesitant to ask for what you want or need.

- What are your plans to improve your assertiveness communication skills?

Boundaries

"Boundaries" refers to the limits we choose in life. It is the process of defining what is acceptable. Boundaries vary between individuals. You define your own boundaries.

Typically, we think of boundaries as being healthy, rigid or blurred. Healthy boundaries are well defined, clearly communicated and respectful to yourself and others. Healthy boundaries are an expression of our identity and although they can change, they generally are stable across time and situations. Changes in boundaries can occur in response to unique circumstances, the environment and people. Our personal experience can lead to a healthy expansion or restriction of a boundary. For example, if you are tired and lonely, a boundary may be that you will not have sex. But once you're in a relationship, given the same circumstances, you may choose to have sex with your partner because of the adult play aspect. While boundaries can change, you should view any rapid changes in your boundaries and limits as a warning sign.

Two types of unhealthy boundaries are blurred and rigid boundaries. They represent the opposite extremes of the spectrum (with healthy boundaries in the middle). Blurred boundaries are too flexible and too changeable. With blurred boundaries, we tend to let the outside environment or other people dictate our beliefs, values and limits. In this situation, we may feel used, violated, exposed and hurt. Our identity is lost. I've experience many clients who think they have a problem because their partner thinks they have a problem.

At the other extreme are rigid boundaries. Rigid boundaries often appear to be extreme stances. In substance-abuse treatment, I talk about an "all or nothing" way of thinking or a "take no prisoners" mentality. The consequences of the rigid boundaries are often isolation, loneliness and judgmentalism.

Three types of boundaries are worth focusing on: *physical, emotional* and *sexual.* Physical boundary is the space around us. When working with children, we use the idea of a "bubble space" surrounding us that intuitively helps children understand how close they can get to another person. The concept of a bubble space supports the idea that boundaries are flexible. Depending on the circumstances, the size of the bubble space changes. For example, we are more comfortable if someone sits next to us in a room full of people, as contrasted with the discomfort we feel when only two people are in the room. Depending on the person and the culture, the bubble space changes as well, and there are different rules on how close you can stand to someone. With friends and family members, our bubble space is smaller; with strangers, it's larger.

Emotional and intellectual boundaries reflect your right to your feelings and thoughts. We individuals have the right to our feelings and beliefs based on values, spirituality, education or cultural affiliation. Our emotional and intellectual boundaries define our personality and identity, and they are a major component in our sexual health. The key is to examine how your boundaries shape your sexual behaviors.

Sexual boundaries reflect your right to your feelings, thoughts and behaviors in the realm of sexuality. We individuals have the right to our feelings and beliefs based on values, spirituality, education or cultural affiliation. These boundaries are a major component in our sexual health. In a future assignment, you will define in detail what behaviors are healthy for you (see page 155).

A boundary violation occurs when someone deliberately or accidentally infringes on the limits of what we are comfortable with. A boundary is violated when you are touched when you do not want to be touched. An emotional boundary is violated when you are subjected to constant criticism, when someone reads another's mail or email without permission, when someone tells us what we should feel or think. The list of potential boundary violations is infinite. In some clients, unhealthy boundaries are a major issue in the recovery process. Using the following list of Signs of Unhealthy Boundaries as a starting place, ask yourself whether any warning symptoms are present. If so, you might be able to trace the symptoms back to a possible boundary violation. Also, ask yourself how the warning symptoms might relate to your sexual health.

Signs of Unhealthy Boundaries

- When you do not want sexual contact, but go along with it anyway so the person will like you.
- Telling someone you like a behavior when you don't.
- Saying you want to get together with someone when you don't.
- Using drugs in a sexual setting when you don't want to.
- Not expressing your sexual desires or preferences with a partner and simply going along with what they want.
- "Falling in love" with anyone who reaches out to you.
- Acting on a first sexual impulse even when you say you will wait until you know the person first.
- Using sex to express anger or loneliness.
- Being sexual for your partner, not yourself.
- Going against personal values to please others.
- Using the Internet as an escape.
- Not noticing when someone else shows poor boundaries.
- Touching a person without asking.
- Letting others tell you what you should or should not do.
- Letting others tell you what is and is not healthy sexual behavior.
- Expecting others to automatically know what you want.
- Engaging in unsafe sex when you say you will not.

Developing healthy boundaries is easier said than done. Learning boundaries is often through trial and error. There is no magic way to develop and express your boundaries. Identifying what you like and dislike is essential. Healthy boundaries are a function of assertive communication where you express your likes and dislikes. It is important that if you don't like something, it's something to communicate and place outside what is acceptable. If you like something, include it within your boundaries. It is your responsibility to express your boundaries to others. As a reminder, this topic serves as a complement to the discussions of Sexual Behavior and Expression (see page 121) and Assertive Communication (see page 110). Please review those discussions again in light of the discussion of Boundaries.

Assignment

- Review your sexual history and timeline. Highlight thoughts, feelings and/or behaviors that might suggest a possible boundary violation.

- Review your sexual history and timeline. What of your boundaries may have been crossed?

- Review your sexual history and timeline. What of other people's boundaries may have been crossed?

- How will you communicate your boundaries to others?

Sexual Behavior and Expression

Sometimes it is easier to explore sexual health issues through a use of a metaphor. A metaphor that I like regarding sexual expression is "ice cream."

Who doesn't like ice cream, one of God's primary gifts to humanity! Imagine, if you will, sitting down with a serving of vanilla ice cream. Think of the creamy feeling, and the taste of vanilla as you eat the first spoonful. Even the frozen vanilla yogurts are good. The soft-serve ice creams are great when you want something in a hurry. Using real vanilla, perhaps with pieces of vanilla beans creates an amazing experience. Some of the premium brands have done a great job making vanilla ice cream almost a spiritual experience! The extra cream makes the texture extra smooth.

Because vanilla ice cream is so good, and so many people like it, I have decided to impose a new rule. Vanilla ice cream in all its variation is the ONLY form of ice cream that is good/holy/sacred. Only vanilla ice cream can be created, served, and sold. I have declared this, so it is.

Absurd, isn't it!

But that is what we've done with sexual expression. Individuals in power eloquently describe why a particular form of sexual expression is good/holy/sacred. Then they impose this value on everyone else.

Absurd, isn't it!

Sexual health requires you to make a choice about what is good/holy/sacred in your life. Yes, you might like "vanilla" but "vanilla" is far from the only flavor of sexual expression. What do you like? Choose.

Historical Definitions of Healthy Sexual Expression

Throughout history, there have been attempts to define sexually appropriate behavior. Within the Judeo-Christian tradition, for example, the "Holiness Code" of the early Israelites was an attempt to define healthy sexual behavior reflecting their values, knowledge and community goals. For a small nomadic people, sexually healthy behavior emphasized procreation. The society's patriarchal system viewed women as property, so most of the holiness code focused on male sexuality. For a society with limited information on biology, the Holiness Code attempted to identify sexually healthy behaviors as a function of blood and energy: loss of blood equaled loss of energy and reflected a threat to survival. As a consequence, women were to be avoided during their menstrual periods.

Fast forward 2000 years to a Europe dominated by the Romans with a new religion (i.e., Christianity) gradually extinguishing paganism. Hence, it was important to reject anything that reflected paganism, including the sexual component of the pagan traditions. Fast-forward another 2000 years – to today and we have a society unlike any previous society, one that understands biology, genetics and multicultural reality. This reality leads to corresponding attempts at defining sexual behavior and a diversity of sexually healthy behaviors.

Many of the historical attempts to define sexual healthy behaviors have emphasized actual sexual acts and condemned the behavior within the context of a religious statement ("This act is unhealthy; it is a sin"). As a result, these definitions are bound by culture and time. Too often individuals are stuck in the trap of asking the "expert" to define what he or she should do. Too often, based on their worldview, clinicians are ready to proclaim what is healthy and what is not.

In the last thirty-five years, experts in the field of human sexuality have attempted to define sexual health. While not reviewed here, the process of defining sexual health has experienced multiple revisions. At one point, scholars argued that a universal definition was not possible given the diversity of people, sexualities, cultures, and circumstances. More recent attempts have attempted to facilitate an interaction between the individual and culture by incorporating a dynamic feedback process in clarifying sexually healthy behaviors. The goal is to help you start thinking about the values that shape your life. As you begin to identify these values, your responsibility is to assess the consistency between these values and your sexual behaviors.

Unhealthy Sexual Behaviors

The consensus among experts in a variety of fields (medicine, mental health, child welfare and clergy) is that only one behavior has consistently been defined as unhealthy: sexual behavior that is exploitive or done without consent. For example, exploitation of children is one of the few universally consistent behaviors condemned across time and across cultures. Yet, even this example has gray areas. In modern America, the definition of a child who can give legal consent for sexual contact ranges from age 14 to age 18. Centuries ago, it was not uncommon for a 12-year-old girl who had just completed puberty (i.e., had a period) to be considered an adult. Today, our collective culture would define this as abuse. Another gray area is exploitation. Activists working against the pornography industry argue that the material exploits women. If so, how does one explain gay pornography? These gray areas highlight the danger and difficulty of universal declarations.

An example sure to raise hackles is the assertion (by a significant group of people) that sexual behavior focused on procreation within marriage is the only form of healthy sex, that any sex act that isn't open to procreation, even within a marriage, is a sin. This approach denounces as sin any form of masturbation or use of pornography. Any sexual behavior is therefore a sin because it doesn't lead to procreation. Some people have modified this approach to emphasize that any sex within marriage is healthy. Still others further modify this approach, believing that any consensual sex within marriage is healthy, recognizing that some traditions emphasize the wife's religious duty to submit to her husband.

Sadly, where to draw the line of healthy vs. unhealthy sexual behavior seems to depend on what side of the line you fall on. If you are "outside" the line, you redraw the line to include your sexual behaviors. Given the relative newness of the Internet, there is a corresponding need for development in defining healthy online behaviors.

Healthy Behaviors

The approach taken in this workbook emphasizes a dynamic process between the community and the individual. Your values determine what behaviors are healthy for you. This is not a do-it-yourself, go-it-alone, I-can-do-anything-I-want. You need your support network. It reflects the community and it is there to provide support, encouragement and accountability. The following is a presentation of four values that are helpful in defining healthy sexual behaviors.

Four values helpful in defining healthy sexual behaviors

Life Giving

The sexual behavior is a positive aspect in your life. This value of sexual behavior is that the experience makes you feel alive and energized. Your personal identity (and your partner's) is affirmed, created and even expanded. You can walk away from the experience with your head held high. There is a sense of fulfillment and even pride in the experience. While life giving, this does not necessarily mean the experience is limited to "great sex" but rather there is an enhancement of identity and personhood for those involved. Sexual behavior is sometimes referred to as "adult play," suggesting a sense of fun, playfulness, and timelessness.

Open and Honest

Healthy sexual behavior is above board, open, and honest. While you may not talk about the incident with everyone because of discretion, you could disclose the activity to your support network. In disclosing to your support network, its members would respond that the behavior is consistent with your declared values and continuing care plan. Not being open and honest is an immediate red flag.

Consent

Full consent and awareness are present in the encounters. Consent implies that all partners are actively giving permission to engage in the behavior, in other words, your not keeping secrets from your support network. Consent requires appropriate disclosures and considerations. This value assumes that full disclosure has occurred with your partner, including risks for STI's, pregnancy, relationship status/availability or statuses your partner should be aware of if the behavior occurs. There is a decided lack of manipulation in the experience. (An example of manipulation is saying, "If you love me, you would have sex with me.")

In some circumstances, consent is not possible. Children are not able to give consent. Relationships with power differences (for example, student/teacher, boss/employee, and therapist/client) are by definition non-consensual. Other circumstances exist where the ability to give consent is questionable because of mental health issues, chemical use or financial status (e.g., "survival sex," where one trades sex for shelter). Another notion embodied within consent is that all parties need to be aware of the experience, which is why exhibitionism and voyeurism are unhealthy - and illegal.

Finally, within the concept of consent is the concept of respect for the partner's boundaries and limits. If consent is removed (i.e., one partner saying "Stop," "No," "I don't want to"), the behavior must stop. Any person can remove consent at any time, with or without a reason.

Responsibility

As a value, responsibility requires that you ultimately assert fully your sexual needs, likes and dislikes. How are you protecting your values? Are the limits you're agreeing to truly yours? Or are they limits you think are necessary because someone else wants you to have them? It is up to you – not the other person – to affirm, communicate and protect your values

Assignment

The following assignment is based on the concept that sexual energy is healthy, and that when it is channeled in healthy ways, it can bring new life and strengthen relationships. Your responses should be harmonious with your values.

Part 1: Review the sex history assignment on page 22. Use this list as a starting point; consider how many of these behaviors are consistent with the four values above in your life. If they are not, remove it from your list of sexually healthy behaviors. Anything that remains is a candidate for a healthy behavior.

Part 2: Answer the following behaviors.

- Who is an appropriate sexual partner for you (age, sex, relationship, etc.)?

- What types of sexual behaviors are healthy for you?

- What types of sexual behavior should you avoid?

- When is it appropriate to be sexually active for you?

- What are healthy reasons to engage in sexual behavior for you?

- What are unhealthy reasons to engage in sexual behavior for you?

- How will you communicate these responses to your partner?

- What do I need to learn about my partner to help my partner experience sexual health?

Chapter 7: Intimacy and Relationships

The majority of most people's life energy is focused on developing connections. In this section, my goal is to help you become aware of the types of intimacy that are important to you, strategize on getting these intimacy needs met and eventually develop the type of relationships that you want.

Desire for Intimacy

One of the best definitions of intimacy is "the feeling of connection with another person. Intimacy is the soul-to-soul connection between two people. Intimacy is a connection with openness and honesty." The need or desire to connect with others is healthy and normal. Most of the memorable moments in our lives are about the experience of intimacy. Similarly, most of the painful memories are about the loss of intimacy. If we look at the present moment, there are many types of intimate connections occurring all the time. Each moment of life is a possible connection to another person. Each moment of life is an experience of intimacy. If we limit our ability to see these intimate connections, then we limit our ability to experience intimacy.

Types of Intimacy

To expand our understanding of intimacy, it is helpful to review different types of intimacy. Once you have reviewed the types of intimacy, the next step is to highlight how to build intimacy in your life. Under each type of intimacy are suggestions on what you might do to enhance your intimacy skills in each area. Use what works for you or develop other ideas. They are far from the only way or the correct way.

Emotional Intimacy

Emotional intimacy is the sharing of significant experiences and feelings. Emotional intimacy is the foundation of all other forms of intimacy. It is the ability to talk without fear. Anything you are afraid of talking about is a possible moment of transformation of fear into intimacy. When fear is present, talking about it can facilitate a stronger and closer relationship. Emotional intimacy includes the ability to share one's hopes and dreams.

- Through therapy, examine life events that have hindered your ability to be in a relationship. These issues might be grief, abuse and/or fear. Share these examples with your support network.

- Read a self-help book. This type of books will help you start to identify and cope with feelings and emotions. Visit a local bookstore and examine titles that speak to you.

- Appropriately share your inner thoughts, feelings, desires and needs with other people in your life.

- Find a support group. Pick a group, such as AA or another program, that addresses an important issue in your life. A wide range of topics exist that may fit your concerns. You'll get a lot of experience sharing your feelings, thoughts, dreams and struggles.

Sexual Intimacy

Sexual intimacy is more than just the physical act of sex. Talking about the deepest and darkest sexual secrets is a form of sexual intimacy. For some of my clients, I am the first individual they talk to about sexuality.

- Attend a workshop on sexuality.

- Share your fantasies with your partner.

- Strategize with your partner about how to make a part (or all) of a fantasy come true (within the rules of your relationship).

- Read a book on sexuality and share with your partner what you liked and disliked.

- Share your work from this workbook with others (as appropriate). Develop plans to get these needs met in ways that are consistent with your life values.

Intellectual Intimacy

Intellectual intimacy is the closeness resulting from sharing ideas. There is a genuine respect for each person's opinion. Agreement on a topic is not required for intellectual intimacy. The process of sharing, reflecting and discussing highlights the aspects of intellectual intimacy.

- Take a class. Check out community colleges, local art groups and area newspapers for classes that may interest you.

- Teach a course.

- Start a book club.

- Join a listserv on a topic of your choice.

- Check out the Internet blogs on a topic of your choice.

Aesthetic Intimacy

Aesthetic intimacy relates to experiences of beauty. This can include expressions of art such as music, plays and movies but also natural beauty such as sunrises, listening to a thunderstorm, and taking a day hike.

- Beauty is definitely in the eye of the beholder, so what do you find beautiful? After you have figured it out, seek it out.

- If you like art, visit a museum, an art space, a play or a movie.

- Love nature? Check out local hiking or outdoor groups to join.

- Missed your shot at "American Idol?" How about joining a local chorus?

- Traditional art not your thing? Walk through your city and photograph graffiti you find interesting. Seek out information regarding body art (tattoos).

- Peruse non-X or R rated Internet sites such as Flickr.

Creative Intimacy

Creative intimacy is the intimacy of shared discovery. The key component is the process of co-creating with another person. Both you and the other person can grow in deeper ways through the experience.

- Bring a friend with you to any activity you enjoy and would like to share.

- Join an art class.

- Read a book on "possibility," such as the *Power of Now* by Eckhart Tolle, or *Power of Intention* by William Dwyer.

Recreational Intimacy

Recreational intimacy refers to the experience of play, stepping beyond the struggles of life and simply spending time together. The types of play include sports, outdoor activities and indoor activities. Sometimes other types of intimacies are incorporated into recreational activities, such as going to a movie (aesthetic) and then talking about it afterward (intellectual).

- Go to the gym, walk or engage in other physical activities.

- Find a club or group to join. For example, most cities have hobby or recreation groups such as bowling or volleyball. Do what you enjoy regardless of what others think. You might be surprised how many people share your interests.

Work Intimacy

Work intimacy occurs in the sharing of tasks. It can include projects, events or the process of long-term commitment regarding work or family. These tasks vary in type, intensity and duration and could include completing a project at work or cleaning up the house. The feeling of satisfaction when completing a task with another person is an example of work intimacy.

- Volunteer for work events or tasks. Join a committee at work.

- Talk with your co-workers about what is going on. As appropriate, ask them what they did last night or over the weekend. Start sharing the basics with them as well.

- Volunteer for organizations or events that are close to your heart. These could be community activities such as a festival or a political campaign.

Crisis Intimacy

Crisis intimacy occurs because of major and minor tragedies. Personal crises may be illness or accidents. Larger forms of crisis intimacy can be community experiences of a natural disaster. In these situations, people step outside of their limits and connect. Strangers will go beyond typical behaviors. The long-term response of the gay community to HIV is a great example of this type of intimacy. The community response to breast cancer is another example.

- Volunteer for a cause that you think is important. This could include rescue missions, food drives and cleanup duty.

- Learn from the crisis and develop long-term safety plans.

Commitment Intimacy

Commitment intimacy is the experience of hope and possibility in response to addressing an issue, cause or event bigger than one individual. This can range from a short-term task (completing a social service project) to a never-ending task such as social justice. It is the process of transforming the world.

- Identify a cause or value that means something to you. Volunteer your time, talent or treasure.

- Within the 12-step tradition, service work is about commitment intimacy.

Spiritual Intimacy

Spiritual intimacy develops through sharing the most important areas of concerns including values, meaning of life and the core of our being. It is an experience of possibility and transcendence beyond the daily experience of who we are. It can include religious traditions and practices, but ultimately it is about how we connect with personal meaning (or with God, in whatever way you understand God).

- Talk to a spiritual advisor of a group different from the one in which you grew up.

- Join a religious faith-group.

- Join a 12-step group. This could be AA but it might also be a 12-step group for partners of AA, Internet sexual compulsivity, debtors, eating and even "Emotions Anonymous."

- Join an online group that discusses life values.

Communication Intimacy

Communication intimacy is the process of full disclosure with another person. It is the process of being open, honest and truthful. This includes giving difficult and constructive feedback, even when it's not easy to do so.

- Simply say what you mean, and mean what you say. (Too often, people say what they think other people want to hear.)

- Learn how to be present and listen to other people by attending a listening training program.

- Continue to share insights into your progress with your support network.

Conflict Intimacy

Conflict intimacy is the process of connecting and respectful fighting, as well as facing differences with others and struggling to understand one another. There is a sense of closeness that transcends conflict and ultimately leads to a closer relationship. The power of "make-up sex" highlights how conflict intimacy is so powerful.

- Recognize that healthy fighting is a normal part of a relationship.

- Learn how to fight in healthy ways by reading a book on conflict manage-ment/resolution, such as *The Eight Essential Steps to Conflict Resolution.*

- Attend an anger-management course.

- Attend a problem-solving course or read problem-solving material online.

The above 12 types of intimacy are simply a place to start. They are not exclusive or exhaustive. Instead, they are designed to help you start thinking of what you want in your life, and how to start getting your needs met in healthy ways. How have you coped with, damaged, or otherwise tried to get these needs met?

Touch/Physical Intimacy

Touch/Physical Intimacy (or Touch Needs) is a form of physical intimacy requiring special focus. The overlap between sexual intimacy and touch intimacy leads to sig-nificant confusion. Classic social psychology research has suggested that the failure to receive touch can have a severe negative health, social and emotional impact on a person. The types of touch exist on a continuum. Nurturing touch is healthy and is expressive of a relationship. Touching people is one way of reaching out and affirm-ing them and being affirmed yourself.

But – at the other end of the continuum – unhealthy touch is the opposite. Exploitive touch is manipulative, forced or unwanted. It can be a way to express hurt, anger or fear. Some touch is confusing; it occurs in the middle or grey area of the touch con-tinuum. In this confusing center are experiences of touch that appear healthy but leave a person unsure about the intent. Examples may be a hug that includes a brush against breasts, buttocks or genitalia, or a kiss that goes on too long. In moving to-ward sexual health, it is important to recognize healthy and unhealthy touch and to identify ways to get your touch needs met. You may also want to review the topic on abuse (see page 81).

In modern American culture, there is a significant barrier to touch. So many of the messages about touch actually sexualize touch. As a result, we may misinterpret the messages of another person. In America, two guys holding hands are seen as a gay couple rather than two friends together, different from the way these two would be viewed in many Middle Eastern cultures. There are also gender differences. Touch is culturally encouraged for many women, but not for men. The typical woman has a better understanding of touch needs than the typical man. The misunderstanding of touch raises significant problems regarding sexual harassment claims. In sexualizing touch, our culture has deprived us of ways to get healthy needs met in appropriate ways. This misunderstanding can lead to miscommunication, conflicts and resentments in sexual, social and emotional relationships.

In developing ways to get your touch needs meet, it is also important to be clear about your motivation. In reviewing your sexual behavior, how many times have you engaged in the behavior when what you were looking for was simply affirmation through touch?

Barriers to Intimacy

Barriers to intimacy can be internal or external. Internal barriers reflect issues in our life and our interaction with others. They may be historical (history of abuse) or current (shame or depression). These barriers can be unhealthy thoughts we have about ourselves or about others. Overcoming, correcting and changing these thoughts is necessary. One example of a person with an intimacy barrier is someone who identifies as a gay man but who believes he is sinful. Another example is an individual who has been abused. These individuals must address the internal story before healthy intimacy is possible. Long-term growth will need to address the fear.

External barriers our outside of ourselves. Examples of these barriers may be isolation or a lack of resources to connect with others. Some of the "-isms" such as sexism, racism, and heterosexism are barriers. With these situations, setting up plans to help you address how the external barriers impact your life can be a helpful approach. Other times the barrier may be a lack of skills that negatively influences a person's ability to communicate with others. In these cases, therapy and coaching may be helpful. You will not find intimacy when you shut down and isolate yourself out of fear. Resorting to the Internet instead of direct, human contact is one way people have figuratively shut down. Intimacy is learned through trial and error. Intimacy sometimes requires the pain of rejection, failure or betrayal. It is not possible to avoid these risks and have intimacy. Your reaction to life's hurts and fears can lead to opportunities for intimacy. The reality is that the other person is probably just as fearful as you are. The question is, which person will be the first to transcend that fear.

Assignment

- As you review your sexual history and your timeline, describe how intimacy (or the lack of intimacy) and sexual behavior relate in your experience.

- What are the messages you have heard about touch from your family, culture, religious tradition or community. How well can you ask others to help with meeting your touch intimacy needs?

- Identify the top three types of intimacy most important to you.

- How would you know if these intimacy needs are satisfied in your life?

- Identify 3–5 people who can help you meet those intimacy needs.

- If you are not satisfied with the type of intimacies, or your level of satisfaction, identify a plan to increase your level of satisfaction.

Dating and Sexual Health

As people start addressing their sexual health issues, eventually they start meeting others, including dating and eventually courtship. Below are eight ideas designed to help frame the desire to date as a process, and a tool for your ongoing journey. Perfection isn't required (or possible), but addressing these concerns will increase your chances for positive experiences.

1. Clarify whether you're ready to date. Dating requires that you have a sense of self, and that you are comfortable in your overall progress. Dating requires assertive communication. It requires that you've defined your basic boundaries including level of disclosure, when disclosure will occur, and a multitude of desires and wants. Examining past dating experiences and addressing triggers that led to relapses is important. One part of this process consists of asking yourself how much you are willing to share about your sexual behaviors. Talking with your support network and addressing their feedback is also important.

2. Clarify your boundaries about which sexual behaviors would be acceptable. Set up explicit boundaries about the type of sexual behavior that can or cannot occur. This needs to be clarified before you start dating.

3. Identify your goals. Be honest with yourself and your support network about what you are looking for in your desire to start dating. Are you looking for friendship?

Sex? Relationship? Children? None of these goals is better than any of the others, but be honest. Develop the skills to effectively communicate these goals with your potential partners. Communicate and get feedback from your support network.

4. Clarify the types of "date" you want. Sometimes starting small is a better plan. You might go on a "coffee date" on a Saturday morning. You might do a lunch date. Instead of calling it a date, describe it as a social chat or a meet-and-greet. Taking the word "date" off the table, and focusing on the social interaction can reduce stress and anxiety. Scheduling it during the day, or mornings (versus Friday evening) can create clarity regarding your goals.

5. Identify activities that you want to do. In identifying your activities, use it to start conversations about what your potential dating partner likes to do. Think outside the box. Review the suggestions on intimacy to consider alternatives to the classic date. You might go to church, go to a museum, go to lecture, etc.

6. Create safety plans. Before you go, make sure you schedule an escape plan, an "out." If you're going for a coffee date, set up an out at 1 p.m. by saying that you have a meeting with a friend at 1 p.m. And set up a meeting with a person from your support network for 1 p.m. to talk about the experience. If the encounter went well, you can always have a second encounter.

7. Remember dating for what dating is. It's a chance to meet and interact with others. You're not making a lifetime commitment to the person on a single date. By addressing the expectations and assumptions you bring to the conversation, you can maintain your focus.

8. Address known concerns beforehand. For example, if you're an introvert develop topics you feel comfortable sharing and asking about. Make sure you are asking questions versus letting the other person set the agenda. If you're the classic extrovert, make sure you listen as well.

For individuals in an existing relationship, it might be helpful to "date" (symbolically) your current partner. Using these ideas may help re-kindle and heal your current relationship.

The Language of Relationships

Much of couples therapy focuses on communication skills. Using the helpful metaphor of language, "undoing the assumption that we all speak the same language" is often the first place of intervention. Consider the following examples. English is the predominant language in the United States, and the assumption is that we all speak English. Yet, even within the United States, different words are used to describe the same concept. For example, New Yorkers enjoying a cola drink might be drinking soda, but Midwesterners enjoying the same drink would be drinking pop. The same holds true in other English speaking countries, like England. Americans on a road trip store their luggage in the trunk of their car, but the Australians store it in the boot. And when the Americans arrive at their destination, they might take the elevator up to their desired floor, but the English might take the lift. Likewise, there are significant differences between Spanish in Latin America and Spanish in Spain. Even Arabic has multiple dialects, and these differences are barriers to communication. So even though people may speak one common language, it is crucial to be aware of differences present in that one common language. Here, we refer to those differences as "dialects." It is important to learn how to understand and translate those dialects.

Similarly, in relationships, it is important to remember that we all have different dialects of communication. These dialects are informed and shaped by the multiple cultures we belong to (age, race/ethnicity, religion, gender, etc.), our family of origin, and our life history. Often, there is enough commonality to be able to communicate with a partner. Most relationship problems stem from communication problems that show up in the guise of unmet expectations and assumptions, hidden wants and needs, past hurts and pains, and hoped for joys and goals.

A classic example is fighting. In some families, conflict is forbidden. A partner learns that anger cannot be expressed. Another partner may come from a family where conflict is resolved quickly and respectfully. When two partners come together, the dialect of conflict is an obstacle to be resolved. The resolution is often as simple as teaching each other their respective dialects. The same idea can be applied to mundane things, like the level of cleanliness in the house, or difficult areas, such as sexual expression, needs and values.

The difficulty in this process is that much of our dialect regarding relationships is automatic and habitual. We assume everyone has the same language, mannerisms, assumptions, and expectations in a relationship. That assumption is often the source of the relationship problems. Teaching each other your individual dialects, and learning to translate your partner's dialect is a necessary skill for building powerful and strong relationships.

Relationship Satisfaction

Relationship satisfaction is a major component of sexual health. As in other topics, sexual behavior can be both a cause, and consequence, of relationship satisfaction concerns. In this topic you are encouraged to focus on your level of satisfaction in your current (or most recent) relationship. Long-term personal happiness, health and wellness are correlated with healthy relationships. One of the more difficult tasks in any relationship is being able to talk with your partner(s) comfortably about sex. The issues can range from simply how often to have sex and or what to do during sex, to whether the relationship should be open, monogamous or some variation thereof.

Respond YES or NO to the following statements:

1. Talking about sex with my sexual partner(s) is a satisfying experience.
2. Overall, I feel satisfied about my current sexual relationship(s).
3. I have difficulty finding a sexual partner.
4. I feel my sexual partner(s) avoids talking about sexuality with me.
5. When I have sex with my sexual partner, I feel emotionally close to him or her.
6. Overall, I feel close with my sexual partner(s).

7.   I have difficulty keeping a sexual partner.

8.   I feel I can express what I like and don't like sexually.

9.   I feel my sexual partner(s) is sensitive to my needs and desires.

10.   Some sexual matters are too upsetting to discuss with my partner(s).

A "yes" response to statements 3 4, 7 and 10 require long-term follow-up. A "no" response to statements 1, 2, 5, 6, 8, 9 require long-term follow-up. Pay attention to the responses that require long-term follow-up. Why did you answer the question the way you did? What are your plans to address the issues raised?

Healing from Past Relationships

When a dog bites a child, there is a high probability that the child will have a negative reaction to dogs in the future. This is an example of transference (see page 35). Any reaction you have to a person is built on your history of experiences. When you have a reaction to a current partner, this reaction is built on your past experiences. When positive, this is helpful. When negative, this can create a barrier that may possibly doom the new relationship.

The amount of hurt arising from past relationships is a major barrier to future relationships. Before you can begin again, you need to clear away the "garbage" of hurt and anger arising from past relationships. Many people will say they are "over" their ex, but our experience suggests otherwise. Review your sexual timeline. How have your past relationships impacted your current sexual behavior and, vice-versa, how has your sexual behavior impacted your relationships? It is important to have a clear understanding about the connection between your life history and your sexual behavior.

It is important to seek help if there are other issues connected to a past relationship. Sometimes the feelings of grief and hurt are so strong, that some type of grief therapy might be important (see page 148). Other issues to consider as possible barriers to future relationships include mental health issues (see page 72), types and impact of abuse (see page 81), stages of identity development (see page 50) or feelings of shame and guilt (see page 44). Until these are addressed, you may be stuck on an escalator trying to go the wrong way.

Forgiveness in Relationships

Forgiveness is not about forgetting. Forgiveness is not about letting the other person off the hook. Forgiveness is about *your* healing. It includes helping you heal from negative thoughts and at the same time helping you let go of painful feelings. It is also an extreme act of compassion when you can forgive the person who hurt you. In some religious traditions, raising forgiveness to a radical expression is offering compassion to the one who offended you. This brings about YOUR radical transformation.

Here are a number of strategies that are helpful in healing from past relationships. They are designed to help create forgiveness in your life.

1. Write a goodbye letter. Share with your support network. Set the letter aside and repeat writing a letter and share again. Repeat again. Keep and review each version. After you've done this 10 times, sit down and review each letter. You will be able to identify a number of themes. And hopefully, you will be able to see your progress in the healing process. Once you have done this about 10 times, if you choose, you may send the 10th version of the letter.
2. Get Support. Reach out to friends, family and professionals.
3. Complete an inventory. Honestly assess your role in the relationship conflict. Step out of the victim role. Recognize that "it takes two to tango." Move forward.
4. Establish a boundary. Despite what your ex might say, your ex's behavior is about your ex, not you. This is important. Remind yourself of it.

Steps in Building the Sexual Relationship

The main goal in any couple's relationship is open and honest communication between partners about what they want, what they don't want and what makes them happy. When your behaviors match your values, it is a sign of sexual health. It is your responsibility to communicate your values to your partner. The degree to which any behavior is consistent with your values is a decision that ultimately rests with you. Regarding sexual expression with your partner, four general tasks are important:

Tell your partner

Have you told your partner what you like and do not like? Too many times, I have run into couples that say to one another, "I didn't know that." For any number of reasons (shame, low self-esteem, fear of being judged, not wanting to upset their partner), individuals will not talk about their likes and dislikes.

Ask your partner

Once you know what you like, you should concentrate on what your partner likes and dislikes. It is important not only to know your partners' likes and dislikes but why he or she has these interests. For example, a couple didn't engage in penetration because it physically hurt. It turned out the pain was due to warts, and once that condition was addressed the problem went away.

Learn

Do not be shy if you do not know how to do something. You may need to learn some basics regarding foreplay, stimulating the clitoris, stretching the vaginal and or sphincter muscle, proper cleanup and so on. You may need to educate your partner.

Get help

If after going through the first three steps you find you are still having problems, you may want to seek some outside help. This does not necessarily mean therapy or counseling, although professional help is a good option for more challenging problems. Try having a frank "out of the box" conversation in which you look at creative outlets and avenues to get your sexual needs met. These could include talking to your spiritual adviser, attending a sexuality workshop or reading various "how to" books. You might go online together to review possible interventions to address the problems. Each of these interventions might be helpful in breaking the logjam in your relationship.

If you have shared your likes and dislikes with your partner and are still having problems, the next steps requires a bit of hard work and honest discussions between you and your partner.

Prioritizing

Some relationships do not focus on sex because they are rich in other ways, such as shared values or emotional connections (see the section on Intimacy, page 123). Consider the importance of your sexual request. Are you willing to live without it? In looking at the whole picture, you might have to agree not to engage in the behavior. This is often the case in "kinkier" types of sexual behavior. In these cases, online sexual behavior might be one way to get these needs met. If you absolutely are unwilling to live without the type of sexual behavior, consider the next two ideas.

Substituting

If your need or desire is important enough that you choose not to live without it, you and your partner need to negotiate an alternative way to get your sexual needs met. This can be difficult, eliciting significant fear, jealousy and raise other issues. It may require changing the type of your relationship (see below).

Transitioning

In my experience, ongoing and significant problems regarding sex can be symptoms of underlying problems within the relationship. While no one likes to hear it, the failure to arrive at a solution might suggest the relationship may not be a healthy one. An example of behavior in an unhealthy relationship might include saying things like "Yes I'll do it" but never intending to follow through. Constantly trying to persuade your partner to engage in a behavior is manipulation and not a healthy sign. A hard and honest look at your relationship may reveal that it is not healthy and that it may need to end. If you are both stuck in this area and don't see a solution, seeking outside professional help may be the best, and possibly the last, option for you.

Relationship parallels for sexual health

Similar to developing sexual health skills, it is also important to develop the corresponding skills in relationship health. In this section, I focus on relationship parallels that you can use to move forward in relationships. As you progress in finding your partner, consider the process it took to even admit or realize you want a relationship. We have mastered the art of skipping over the tough, ambiguous parts of life – now we are learning to navigate the unknown, vulnerable, exhilarating process of life. Consider the guide below as you put yourself out into the dating world.

1. Looking. Physical attraction or that "something" about the other person is often what first sparks interest, but to what else are you attracted? How important is it that your partner demonstrate values consistent with yours? Do you want someone with whom you can laugh? Is intellectual stimulation important to you? What about openness? Is it important to have a partner who is friendly, polite, compassionate, and/or sincere? Consider other general characteristics that you wish to have in a partner. It may also be helpful to consider to what extent you yourself demonstrate these qualities. If you need to, set rules for yourself. Some rules may be the following: no naked times until at least (pick a number) months have passed, no overnight dates until at least (pick a number) dates, no sex until you really know (and still like) the person. Also consider your non-negotiables: he/she must be gay/bi/etc. and un-partnered and out, he/she must have (pick a time period) length of sobriety and/or not use, he/she must demonstrate general levels of respect, social decorum, etc. Finally, reflect on what have you struggled with in the past and what are you intent on changing?

2. Chatting/Flirting. In the early stages of dating or getting to know someone, you are doing just that – getting to know a person. You are getting to know him and how you are or how you feel when you are with him. Does he/she interest you? Does he/she laugh with you, or do your jokes fall on seemingly deaf ears? Does he/she make fun of people rather than use humor in a non-destructive way? When you are in the chatting stage, you are at the beginning stages of getting to know someone. Generally, topics of conversation involve current events, pop culture, likes and dislikes, general relationship histories or life lessons. This is the "hanging out" period, so consider playing and having fun. Face to face contact is probably once per week and maybe a chat or two during the week. Notice and heed what is comfortable for you. And remember: you are dating and getting to know the person. You aren't married yet.

3. Spending more time together. As you get to know each other, you increase the time you spend together. If things are going well, this is when you might start thinking: will we want dogs or cats, does he want kids, or where will the honeymoon be? Re-

sist judging the fantasies as good or bad, or trying to "figure out" if he likes you as much. Just note that they are fantasies and reconnect with the moment and stage of the relationship. If you were dating others when you met, you are likely both still dating other people; but you may begin to notice that you are particularly fond of this one.

4. Emotional touching. When you begin to notice that you are really happy when he/she texts or calls or you feel noticeably excited to see him, you have progressed to the "emotional touching" phase. You likely exchange confessions of "I like you," "you're cool," etc. You begin to experiment with the idea of progressing to a true, "I'm interested in you" dating relationship. Questions of "where is this going" or questions of a celestial nature are answered in the interaction itself. If you are wondering how he/she feels about you, consider his actions: does he seem happy to see you, do you talk, is the interaction balanced? Trusting yourself is key and takes practice. Notice the state of your anxiety level – this may be when you typically would have either bolted or started really worrying about whether the other person likes you, or when you typically start covertly criticizing him or her. Pause, regroup and stay focused on yourself (yes, attend to the interaction, but remember it is not just about the other person – if the other person doesn't call you back for 5 days, fine – this is about you practicing being grounded and authentic). Check in with yourself, how do you feel with the other person? Do you feel good and energized? Do you feel uncharacteristically dominant or uncharacteristically submissive or uncharacteristically somewhere in the middle? Periodically, ask yourself these questions.

5. Emotional Petting. Ok, so you really like each other. You really like the other person. Notice the stirrings you feel. Remember to take care of yourself during this time. Keep working, keep spending time with your other friends and family. Yes, feel excited about your new guy or gal, but continue to attend to yourself. As you continue to get to know the relationship, ask yourself whether you would be proud to introduce him or her to your friends and family. Have you met his or her friends and family? If you have done this already, how did it go? If you haven't done this and have wanted

to, consider what is happening (e.g., are you nervous or noticing "red flags")? Do you feel comfortable having a conversation about this?

6. Full Heart Touching. As the relationship progresses, you will feel more of a connection. You will share more of your histories, etc. Be mindful when sharing your story. You are not "hiding" parts of yourself or your past. This is not about shame or keeping secrets; rather, you are learning about, setting, and experiencing your emotional and psychological boundaries. Do not assert more vulnerability than you are willing to lose. For example, if you feel a rush to disclose something or if you are anxious to inquire about the other person's response to more details of your history, notice what happens (your internal dialogue) or what you are thinking about before you take the plunge. This is not to say, "don't do it," just have a sense of your goals or hopes in doing it.

Be equally mindful when hearing the other person's story. Is the person going too fast for you? What is the person "pulling from" or touching in you? For example, does the person talk in detail about how much he or she has been hurt and do you feel the need to take care of him or her, or does the person assert anger about someone to the point where you start to feel nervous? Does the person "push" you or ask you questions you are not ready to answer? Does the person respect your boundaries when you set them? Notice what is happening within yourself: is it feeling too close? Are you changing yourself in some way? How can you correct this?

7. True Vulnerability. You have decided "it is the two of you," and things are going well. You know the other person as a separate being. You get who the other person is, quirks and all; and the other person gets you, quirks and all. The intimacy progresses to different levels, you feel like you have a close friend or partner with the other person. You are your best self.

8. Mutual Expression. You can talk with each other about everything: values, spirituality, family, work, friends, sex, likes and dislikes, whether to have an open or not open relationship and related expectations. Although the connectedness and openness is there, you are still psychologically and emotionally autonomous. You have your

bad days still but you know your partner is not responsible for not anticipating your every need. You still take care of yourself, but you have a supportive partner.

9. No more Fantasy Land. Believe it or not, part of healthy relationships includes conflict at times. This is not about "I want Thai and he wants Burger King," this is a fight where you might hurt each other's feelings, say things you shouldn't, etc. When you take time to look at the conflict notice how you experience it: do you feel victimized, do you feel he/she was "totally" in the wrong, are you thinking of ending it? What is happening in your world? Consider how the fight emerged, what happened? What was it about? Did it involve others? Were you starting to feel anxious and restless? Did you "pick" the fight? Did he or she "pick" the fight? Was there a need that hadn't been met or stated? Consider the content of the fight and the process of the fight. The other person has disappointed you and you have disappointed the other person. You are both totally human. How will the relationship tolerate this?

10. Break-through (first kiss and make up). How did you resolve the conflict? Resolution takes time. Re-attuning with your partner is something of a process, depending on the nature, intensity and frequency of the conflict. Do you feel good about how the resolution occurred? Did you both consider each other's feelings and person? Did you just feel blamed? Were you really blamed or was that an internal conversation (review the discussion on mindfulness on page 35) and were you able to discuss the internal messages with your partner? Did you feel you both worked at it and met in the middle?

Often, a conflict of sorts brings couples closer, provided the conflict is "fair." In working through the conflict, you both describe only your own positions (no one is the victim and no one is the abuser). This means you are grounded in your own experience. If you have a guess as to the other person's reality, then ask, but you cannot read the other person's mind — he/she is doing what makes sense to him/her and you are doing what makes sense to you. What can you learn from the conflict? For example, if one person was starting to feel resentful about something, how assertive were each of you? At the same time, where was the other person and did he/she know? Now repeat steps 1-10 multiple times.

11. Transformation. You have the house in the Hamptons and a pet tiger (now keep repeating steps 1-10 in no particular order…and remember to keep playing and having fun).

Type of Relationships

Culture is very powerful in shaping our view of what is a healthy relationship (see Culture and Stereotypes on page 36). Our current culture emphasizes that sexual behavior should occur within a monogamous relationship, and that only monogamous relationships are healthy. How much do you agree with this expectation? In fact, there are a multitude of different types of relationships. Sexual health requires that you clarify the type of relationship you want. This is a controversial area, and clinicians legitimately differ in their opinions. The primary approach taken in this book is that you have the responsibility to choose the type of life you want to live regarding sexual expression. There is a vast amount of material written on relationships. As a summary, I highlight three types of sexual relationships:

Celibacy and Singledom

Celibacy is often confused with singledom, but it is different. Definitions vary, but I define celibacy as a choice not to engage in any sexual contact with anyone. There are opinions saying that any sexual expression including masturbation, fantasy and use of sexually explicit material go against the idea of celibacy. Other opinions say that celibacy does not allow any genital contact with a person. Some religious traditions impose celibacy as the only form of sexual expression for groups of people (usually LGBT individuals or non-married straight couples). Also, some religious traditions impose celibacy as a discipline in order for a person to qualify to be a minister in that tradition.

Rightfully understood, however, celibacy is less about telling yourself "you can't do that" than about emphasizing something greater in a person's life. Celibacy allows a greater commitment to the major focus in a person's life. In this approach, celibacy is believed to facilitate other types of intimate relationships (see Types of Intimacy on page 123). In my opinion, a healthy expression of celibacy is possible. It does take work and self-understanding. And celibacy doesn't "turn-off" the sexual energy within a person. If you choose this, you *must* find *healthy* ways to channel your sexual energy. It is very important to choose celibacy for the right reason. I've run into many individuals who "choose" celibacy out of fear, a history of abuse, or low self-esteem. If these are the motivating factors for choosing celibacy, it is only a matter of time until a commitment or vow of celibacy will be broken.

Singledom is the choice to remain single and not be in a relationship. Often, people do not consider singledom as a choice, given the assumption from the primary culture that everyone should be in a relationship. The pressure toward coupling is profound and subtle. Watch what happens with your couple-friends when you break up a relationship. Think about Grandma's first comment when you go home for the holidays: "Have you found someone yet?" It is an expression of concern for your happiness, but it does demonstrate the social pressure toward coupling, and it implies that something is wrong with remaining single. Singledom is simply an option on how to live out your life. It may, or may not, include celibacy. It may be short or long term. It is simply a choice. As in all other choices, the reason that you are choosing to be single is the key question for you. Understanding your motivations (including perhaps some of the unspoken reasons) is a key to sexual health.

Monogamy

Monogamy is typically defined as sexual contact exclusively between two individuals within some type of committed relationship. Even this definition has different interpretations, resulting in confusion and conflict. For some people, monogamy is expanded to prevent any emotional relationships with anyone but the primary partner. Some interpretations of monogamy also view use of sexually explicit material as a violation of monogamy. So, for some couples, online sexual behavior would be a violation of the commitment to monogamy, but in other couples, this would be okay. The key is for you and your partner to clarify your opinions.

Healthy monogamy is about trust and commitment. It means working with your partner to put the other first. And – paradoxically in putting the other first, your needs are met, in part because your partner is putting you first. Monogamy isn't passive; it requires tremendous amounts of work. This book is designed to start the necessary conversations regarding healthy monogamy, to make it possible for you to choose monogamy for the right reasons. When monogamy is chosen out of fear, it is less about an expression of love than an expression of fear and attempted control over your partner. There is a decided lack of trust. (The same concerns exist in choosing any type of relationship. When chosen out of fear, it probably is not a healthy choice.)

Open/Poly Relationships

Open relationships are typically defined as a relationship where there exists a primary sexual and emotional partner followed by a secondary partner or partners. (Given the focus of the book, there isn't the space to fully address poly relationships and alternative relationships. For more information, read *Ethical Slut* by Easton and Litsz or check out www.xeromag.com as one example). Within the concept of open/poly relationships, there are a variety of definitions and expressions. If you choose an open relationship it is important for you and your primary partner to clarify ground rules and expectations. When, where, with whom and how often are all topics to be addressed. What are the plans for communicating and coping with fear, jealousy and insecurity? What are the safer-sex rules?

If you want an open relationship, examine what unmet needs (if any) exist within your primary relationship. Significant reflection should occur within your support network to clarify the reasons you want an open relationship. In particular, be careful that you are not simply trying to get out of the primary relationship. If the primary relationship is not healthy, it is important to address the issues first. If it should end, do this with integrity instead of forcing a rift that ends the relationship. One guideline is that all partners be open and honest in the conversation. Both partners must agree with a sense of internal integrity with any decision. It might be better to end a relationship than agree to a type of relationship that is inconsistent with your values.

Sexual satisfaction is a major component of overall relationship satisfaction. Research has repeatedly stressed that overall health is connected to relationship satisfaction. If you continue to struggle in this area, I strongly recommend seeking additional help from a qualified professional.

Assignment

- Review your sexual timeline and relationship history for any patterns. Was your behavior in response to something your partner did? Was your partner's behavior in response to something you did? If so, describe the details?

- If applicable, what plans do you need to include for ongoing healing?

- Clarify what type of relationship you want in your life. Explain this to your support network. Review this with your partner.

- Review the topic on Sexual Behavior and Expression (see page 104). What type of sexual behaviors do you enjoy? Share these with your partner.

- Review the same list and ask your partner what he or she likes?

- Review your relationship history. If there are any unhealed relationships (see page 136), identify plans to address the past relationship(s).

- What are your primary barriers to a healthy relationship?

- Identify plans to address the concerns raised by each of these questions.

Feelings of Grief

Grief is an issue sometimes connected with sexual health concerns and in particular relationship history. Various theories have explained the process of grief. I like best the model presented by Elizabeth Kübler-Ross, who identified five stages of grief: denial, anger, bargaining, depression and acceptance.

As others have also done, I've made a few tweaks to Kübler-Ross's model to include the role of perceived losses, the role of small losses and the "time focus" of grief. Feelings of grief typically result from a significant loss, such as a death of a loved one, but grief from other losses can also have a powerful impact on a person's life. Take, for instance, the end of a relationship or friendship, or the loss of a job. Grief may also be due to the loss of hopes, dreams or fantasies. For example, in a gay person's coming-out process, the person may feel a loss, because recognizing a same-sex identity ends the perception of a "normal" life. Sometimes, the symbolic meaning of an event, location or person triggers an experience of loss. Moving from your home results in recognition of the end of a sense of security. These perceived losses could have the same impact as a tangible loss.

Some feelings of grief are anticipatory; in this situation, you might foresee the end of something. This may show up as "This is a bad relationship; I need to get out of it, so I go online, I can avoid having to deal with the bad relationship."

One of the critiques of Kübler-Ross's model is the perception that the process of coping with grief is linear; you simply go from one stage to the next. I think grief is cyclical; you might see the parts of a stage a number of times. You may move from acceptance back to denial, etc. I believe the key is to recognize that, whatever the situation, it is acceptable and healthy to be present when experiencing your thoughts and feelings.

A second critique of the Kübler-Ross model is the implication that process occurs once and is rather quick. It is important to remember that coping with a loss takes awhile. In some circumstances, the grief process can last a year or more. In addition grief can be triggered when certain rituals, anniversaries or memories occur. Our culture often minimizes the long-term impact of grief.

A third critique is that the model focuses only on "negative" feelings, failing to honor the positive feelings that can accompany the process. It isn't uncommon to rapidly cycle from sadness, to happiness to anger, and back to relief.

As you review your sexual history, pay attention to how the following stages of grief may have played out. A few examples describe how people might experience the stage.

Stages of Grief

Denial

The goal in this stage is to avoid dealing with the intensity of the grief. This can include actively avoiding the grief or minimizing the loss. Behaviors in this stage include not talking about the loss, glossing over it, or providing a minimal response to avoid further discussion such as "I'm fine" or "It's no big deal."

Anger

In this stage, the energy around coping with grief goes outward. The person may feel victimized or attacked. "This isn't fair." Statements regarding men might include "All men are like that."

Bargaining

In this stage, there is recognition of grief, but the coping mechanism leads one to minimize the impact of grief. A person might begin dating before the grief is resolved (a rebound relationship). Another way this may be present is selecting a new partner with the thought that "He or she is better than no one" or "He or she isn't like the last one." Or, still, "I'll just go online so I don't get hurt."

Depression

Common thoughts in this stage include "Why try?" "Nothing matters" or even "It will never get better." One of the difficulties in distinguishing between depression and grief is that depression is part of the grief process. Review the discussion of depression (see page 74). Might any of the depression symptoms you're experiencing be related to grief?

Acceptance

By this point, you integrate grief into your life, and while grief may be present, it has lost most of its intensity. This means you can acknowledge the loss, but the loss does not result in a barrier to healthy relationships or daily functioning. In some cases, the loss may actually facilitate transformation. These are signs of successful adjustment to grief.

Assignment

- Describe circumstances when you've felt feelings of grief. How has this related to your sexual behavior (is the grief a consequence of the behavior, or is grief a cause of the behavior)?

- When you find yourself feeling grief, what other feelings may be associated with the grief?

- What are your plans to improve your ability to express grief in healthy ways?

Finding a relationship therapist

Finding a couple's therapist, or a relationship therapist, is important, but it can be difficult. A juggling metaphor in relationship therapy helps to demonstrate the challenge of relationship therapy. At the start of relationship therapy, there are three balls to juggle: Person A, Person B, and the Relationship. The "three balls" of relationship therapy make creating change in the relationship more difficult than individual therapy. Realistic expectations about timing and progress are important.

Before you start, to the best of your ability clarify your goal. While it might be hard to acknowledge, if you know that you don't want to stay in the relationship, be honest up front for the sanity of everyone. This includes your sanity, your partner's sanity and the clinician's sanity.

Many times the individuals in the relationship will start therapy during a rocky period. If either one of the individuals is unsure about the future of the relationship, your therapist may ask for a time commitment from both of you to discern your intentions and to work on the relationship.

Remember that the RELATIONSHIP is the client, not the individuals. Most individual therapists will NOT do relationship therapy when working with one member of the relationship. There are appropriate exceptions, so this is not an absolute rule. Check with the therapist.

During the intake session, put everything on the table, whether it is sexual issues, insecurity, jealousy, communication, respect, or whatever. Often, the second and third sessions are individual meetings to provide each individual an opportunity to put additional issues on the table that may be too difficult in the first session, such as sexual contact outside the primary relationship. Sharing everything is important. For example, if you engage in alternative sexual behaviors, or if you had a sexual contact outside the relationship, say so.

Chapter 8: Spirituality, Values and Sexual Health

This section addresses spirituality and sexual health. I am very supportive of religious traditions. There are some tremendous sexual health values taught by many religious traditions. But I also recognize that too often in sexuality, religious messages may actually be a barrier to sexual health. A journey toward sexual health may require alternatives to a religious tradition. For many, the concept of a higher power is helpful. Nevertheless, a common theme in both religious and spiritual traditions is recognition of the importance of core values that shape your life. I end this section by identifying strategies that you can use to help in your process of identifying the core values that you use to define your personal definition of sexual health.

In many ways, spirituality can shape and focus our values, goals and behaviors. The goal for this section is to help you clarify how consistent your values are concerning sexual behavior.

I distinguish between religion and spirituality. The distinction reflects the difference between the individual and the community. "Spirituality" reflects *your* faith, values, and experiences of the holy. "Religion" reflects the *community's* faith, values and experiences of the holy. The two are different but related.

It is through one's experience of spirituality that one connects with a community of faith. To develop one's spirituality, it may help to review your understanding of scripture and tradition, to create a positive approach to morality and higher power. Scripture and tradition are not always an enemy to spirituality. Within a tradition, a sense of wholeness and acceptance is possible. Tradition expresses a community's experience of "God" or "The Holy." This is true whether it is a long-term tradition (such as Jewish, Christian, Muslim, Catholic, Buddhist traditions) or a newer tradition (such as fellowship after a 12-step group).

Barriers to Spirituality

Three barriers to spirituality are religiosity, fundamentalism and lack of education. Consider how these barriers may be present in your life.

Religiosity is based on the performance of duties without the integration of spiritual values. Early on, I discussed the need for integrity (see page 10). Many individuals profess a faith but fail to live by that faith. Their behavior is focused on appearances, on looking good, and using religion as a means of looking good. The number of public sex scandals by those who profess a religious tradition proves this point. In emphasizing a healthy life, many religious traditions actually suppress sexuality versus finding healthy outlets. Religiosity is one means of suppressing sexuality.

Fundamentalism occurs in two primary ways: scriptural fundamentalism and dogmatic fundamentalism. Essentially, fundamentalism sets up a thinking error that one view of scripture or belief is the only right view. This creates a series of judgments about who qualifies as a person of faith. Fundamentalism dictates only a narrow manner in which faith can be expressed. In an attempt to help people, the fundamentalist approach usually results in excluding many people.

Lack of education is a final barrier. Many people simply have too little education in their faith tradition to begin the process of uncovering the richness of that tradition. Not many individuals can explain the dogmas and doctrines that can provide a rich resource for future growth.

As you move toward increased spiritual health, it might be helpful to address any struggles you have had with fundamentalism or with feeling judged and rejected. It may also be helpful to increase your education within your tradition. Addressing your struggles and increasing your education might help affirm your sexual health and clarify your values.

Power of Story

The process of developing spirituality is to recognize the importance of "story." Spirituality starts and ends with a theology of story. This is a process where we identify experiences of God. (For convenience, I use the term, "God," but included are such terms as, "Higher Power," "Goddess," "Spirit," "Wisdom," "The Absolute," "The "All," etc.) A theology of story helps us recognize that scripture is simply a collection of stories of people's experiences of God. Typically, these oral stories were written down, collected and made official across time. In other words, a person had an experience of God, and then shared the experience with another person who was also so inspired that he shared it with others. People wrote down and collected these stories. This collection eventually became what we see as "scripture."

The application of a theology of story to our daily life is important. A theology of story asks, "What experiences of God in my life have I encountered?" It is in recognizing these experiences that we begin the process of seeing how God is present in our life. The difficulty is that we have lost the ability to share new stories. Many people deny their experiences of the holy. Furthermore, because of fundamentalism, scriptures have unfortunately become a basis to condemn people instead of being a collection of people's experience of God. The use of scriptures as a weapon has led to difficulty in sharing our personal stories.

Part of the process of developing your spirituality is to understand how we experience God in various ways by discussing three approaches to developing spirituality: **positive spirituality, generativity** and **creative mythology**. Each can give you insight into your own story of God experiences. **Positive spirituality** emphasizes a process of uncovering the values by which you choose to live your life. It is future oriented. We make decisions and express our values as a reflection of our experience of God. Positive spirituality focuses on goals or values such as wholeness, integrity, fidelity and growth that a person seeks to express. For those with a religious tradition, the values we choose to live by can come from our community experience. Many values identified in the scriptures and traditions are positive. Examples include love, integrity, forgiveness and responsibility. These values shape our life. A typical example of this is the WWJD ("What Would Jesus Do?") bumper sticker. A person with a WWJD sticker has declared "As a Christian, who believes in Jesus, I use His life to shape my behavior as an expression of my beliefs."

Positive spirituality is future focused, but **generativity** focuses on the now. Generativity asks the question, "How am I being made whole in the now?" In other words, in this experience (or with this thought) "Am I brought to a sense of wholeness, or am

I left distracted and broken. In the realm of sexual health, does this behavior help or hinder my well-being?"

The concept of **creative mythology** is based on research by Joseph Campbell. For him, creative mythology focuses on how people express meaning in their lives. He says creative mythology is "present when an individual has an experience of order, horror, beauty, exhilaration, which seeks to be communicated through signs, images, and words."

Campbell's research suggests that a focus on the experience of something amazing, either good or bad, shifts an individual's understanding of reality, and that in these experiences a person connects to God. Then, the person shares his experiences with other people. Creative mythology is an attempt to identify and express meaning of something greater in a person's life by noticing these important experiences. Mythology is a way one person's heart speaks to another person's heart. Notice the similarity between creative mythology and the concept of intimacy, as discussed in the topic Intimacy (see page 123).

Assignment

This assignment will help you to start thinking about something greater in your life. Think "big" about your future. What would a "life you love" look like? Spirituality requires you to make a commitment to take responsibility in your life. You need to step forward to identify and claim the values that you find important, the values that you will use to shape your life. What works for some people will not necessarily work for you. We may learn from each other, but our paths are uniquely our own.

- Identify three people who inspire you. These people may be real or fictional, living or dead, someone you know, or simply someone you've read about. For each person, identify why this person is an inspiration to you. Examine two or three values this person has expressed through his or her life. As you think about each person, you may start to identify themes that are important to you.

- Name three times when you experienced a sense of timelessness. Some authors describe this as "being in the flow". In this context, "timelessness" is the experience of time passing without your awareness. Think of a young child playing outside all day. You say to the child, "Come in for bed." To the child, the day passed with a sense of timelessness. They simply were completely in the moment. Describe the settings in which you experienced timelessness, focusing on who, what, when, and where. What words do you use to summarize how these experiences inspire you?

- As you examine the individuals and experiences in your life that are important, make note of common themes, values and experiences. These themes are expressions of your experience of God in your daily life.

- After listing the themes, review each word in a dictionary or Wikipedia. Learn the depth of meaning of these words. Summarize what you learn.

List three to five values that express your spirituality. Below are some examples. These values are broad and primarily evoke a calling to move beyond the big and little fears of life and step into a greater life. In the field of morality, we might label these values as virtues. Find the values that inspire you. Examples of possible values include the following. (If you find one that you like, continue to research the term.)

Justice

Justice is often reduced to holding people accountable, sort of like a punishment. This is a start, but justice is also about restoring a sense of harmony and connection. Justice is more than just fairness; it's also about the common good.

Peace

Peace is the absence of conflict, but it also includes the ideas of harmony, connection and common purpose. Peace also refers to a sense of internal purpose, being grounded and a sense of internal acceptance. Within the concept of peace is a connection to justice.

Generosity

Generosity is often seen as giving to others on a monetary level. Generosity can also include giving of talent and time. Included are the concepts of focusing on others and the common good. Generosity is giving someone the benefit of the doubt by interpreting comments and statements from a view toward growth instead of failure.

Love

Love often focuses on a strong emotional attachment. The English understanding of Love is based on the term "charity," which can include a sense of unconditional acceptance of another person.

Wisdom

Wisdom is more than intelligence; it's the application of experience with knowledge. Within the concept is a sense of integrity and being grounded. Applying wisdom creates justice. Wisdom can also include leading by experience.

Compassion

Compassion is about caring for others. It includes the profound understanding of another's experience. It's about entering into a conversation with a willingness to understand another person's point of view, even if you disagree. Compassion calls forth justice and wisdom.

Courage

Courage includes the concept of bravery. It's not just about acting without fear; it's also about acting through fear. You will experience fear moving forward; courage is about continuing to move forward. Sharing everything with your support network is an example of courage. Courage primarily occurs when you face a struggle or challenge.

Integrity

Integrity requires a level of self-awareness and commitment to live according to the inner truth. This means saying what you mean, and meaning what you say. Honoring your word is a major part of integrity. Integrity occurs when your behaviors and values are consistent with one another.

Your Values

Your task is to identify values that are important to you. Ask yourself how your values shape your behaviors, your limits, your response to fears and your boundaries. Does a particular sexual behavior move you closer or further away from your values? Our experience suggests that when we are living lives based on our values, we are living lives we love.

The challenge is to ask yourself, "How willing am I to do whatever it takes to express my values in living?" Our inspirations are often people who, despite their fear, choose actions that express their values. Think of people such as Martin Luther King Jr., Gandhi and Mother Theresa. They expressed their values in their daily lives to the degree that the world recognized them as inspiring.

The values that inspire you are remarkably stable, yet they can sometimes change. More often it is our awareness, language and skill in understanding and expressing our values that change, more than our values themselves. Please pay attention to both the typical meaning as well as the philosophical meaning of the values that are most important to you. Value clarification is a continuing process — a process, not a product. You can use your values to shape your continuing-care plan in a profound way. The key questions are, "Will this behavior protect my values?" and "How do my values shape the next step for me?"

Using the values listed above – justice, peace, generosity, love, wisdom, compassion, courage and integrity – simply as starting points with the addition of any other values you identified, the five values that are most important to you are:

1.

2.

3.

4.

5.

A New Beginning: Continuing the Conversation

The next step...

Now that you have finished the workbook, use the values from the previous page and review your responses throughout the workbook. Are your values expressed in your responses? If so great; if not great. What is left is to start again. In the process, you can gain a deeper awareness of what you need to express a life you love. My experience is that individuals have new levels of understanding when they review past assignments. Ongoing analyses of these assignments may provide insight into creating a new breakthrough. Repeating assignments may allow new understanding of previously forgotten materials or new understanding of your relationships. A decrease in feelings of shame may allow you to deal with a deeper secret not previously shared.

SexualHealthInstitute.blogspot.com

Much of the material in this workbook I posted in draft form on my website via the blog, http://sexualhealthinstitute.blogspot.com. After completing the workbook, the blog became a place to add material, provide reactions and comments and a starting point for conversation. Please feel free to review the blog for new material. You are encouraged to suggest ideas, ask questions, or participate in any way you feel comfortable. For the safety of all, I moderate all posts. All posts are anonymous unless you give me explicit permission to use your name. Questions and instructions to consider:

- What has been helpful?
- What topic would you want more information about?
- Is there a missing topic?
- As you develop your sexual health, what have been your greatest struggles?
- Share examples of success.
- Describe areas where things fell apart.

Additional Resources

The following resources reflect most of the material used in the writing of the book. (I've been doing this nearly 20 years, and don't always remember where I read something) I am grateful to my colleagues, known and unknown who have taught me so much.

Ackard, D & Kearney-Cooke, A. (2000) Effect of Body Image and Self-Image on Women's Sexual Behaviors. *International Journal of Eating Disorders, 28(4)*, 422-429.

Baird, Robert J. (2004) Clergy and cybersex: A motivational study. Ph.D. dissertation, Union Institute and University, United States , Ohio. Retrieved March 9, 2011, from Dissertations & Theses: Full Text. (Publication No. AAT 3157507).

Bancroft, J. & Vukadinovic, Z. (2004) Sexual Addiction, Sexual Compulsivity, Sexual Impulsivity, or What? Toward a Theoretical Model. *Journal of Sex Research, 41(3)*, 225-234.

Bean, J. (2002) Expressions of Female Sexuality. *Journal of Sex & Marital Therapy. Supplement 1, 28(1)*, 29-38.

Brick, P. (1991) Fostering Positive Sexuality. *Educational Leadership, 49(1)*, 51-53.

Bockting, W., Rosser, S. & Scheltema, K (1999) Transgender HIV prevention: implementation and evaluation of a workshop, *Health Education Research, 14(2)*, 177-183, doi: 10.1093/her/14.2.177

Carballo-Diéguez, A., Miner, M., Dolezal, C., Rosser, S. & Scott, J. (2006). Sexual negotiation, HIV-status disclosure, and sexual risk behavior among Latino men who use the Internet to seek sex with other men. Archives of Sexual Behavior, 35, 473-481.

Carnes, P. (1992) *Out of the shadows.* Center City, MN: Hazelden.

Carnes, P. (1997) *Sexual anorexia.* Center City, MN: Hazelden.

Carnes, P., Delmonico, D. L. & Griffin, E. (2001) In the shadows of the net: Breaking free from compulsive online sexual behavior. Center City, MH: Hazelden Foundation Press.

Cass, V. (1984) Homosexual Identity Formation: Testing a Theoretical Model. *Journal of Sex Research, 20(2)*, 143-167.

Clinebell, H. & Clinebell, C. (1970) *The Intimate Marriage* Harper & Row.

Coleman, E. (1991) Compulsive sexual behavior: New concepts and treatments. *Journal of Psychology and Human Sexuality, 4*(2), 37-52.

Coleman, E. (1992) Is your patient suffering from compulsive sexual behavior? *Psychiatric Annals, 22*(6), 320-325.

Coleman, E. (2002) Masturbation as a means of achieving sexual health. *Journal of Psychology & Human Sexuality, 14(2-3)*, 5-16. doi:10.1300/J056v14n02_02

Coleman, E. (1995) Treatment of compulsive sexual behavior. In R. Rosen, & S. R. Leiblum (Eds.), *Case studies in sex therapy* (pp. 333-349). New York, NY: Guilford Press.

Coleman, E., Raymond, N. & McBean, A. (2003) Assessment and treatment of compulsive sexual behavior. *Minnesota Medicine, 86(7)*, 42-47.

Coleman, E. (1995) Treatment of compulsive sexual behavior. In R. Rosen, & S. R. Leiblum (Eds.), *Case studies in sex therapy* (pp. 333-349). New York, NY: Guilford Press.

Cooper, A., Delmonico, D. L. & Burg, R. (2000) Cybersex users, abusers, and compulsives: New findings and implications. *Sexual Addiction & Compulsivity*, 7(1-2), 5-29. doi: 10.1080/10720160008400205

Cooper, A., Delmonico, D. L., Griffin-Shelley, E. & Mathy, R. M. (2004) Online sexual activity: An examination of potentially problematic behaviors. *Sexual Addiction & Compulsivity*, 11(3), 129-143. doi:10.1080/10720160490882642

Corley D & Schneider (2002) *Disclosing Secrets: When, to Whom and How Much to Reveal* Gentle Path Press.

Co-Sex Addicts Anonymous (COSA) http://www.cosa-recovery.org/

Cotton, M. Ball, C. & Robinson, P. (2003) Four Simple Questions Can Help Screen for Eating Disorders *Journal General Internal Medicine*, 18(1): *53–56*.doi: 10.1046/j.1525-1497.2003.20374.x.

Daneback, K., Cooper, A. & Månsson, S. (2005) An Internet study of cybersex participants. *Archives Of Sexual Behavior, 34(3)*, 321-328.

Deacon, S. & Minichiello, V. (1995) Sexuality and older people: Revisiting the assumptions. *Educational Gerontology, 21(5)*, 497-513.

Dekker, A & Schmidt, G. (2002) *Patterns of Masturbatory Behaviour: Changes Between the Sixties and the Nineties.* Co-published simultaneously in *Journal of Psychology & Human Sexuality*. 142/3, 35-48; and: Masturbation as a Means of Achieving Sexual Health (ed: Walter O. Bockting and Eli Coleman) The Haworth Press, Inc., 35-48.

Demarest, J. & Allen, R. (2000) Body Image: Gender, Ethnic, and Age Differences *Journal of Social Psychology, 140(4)*, 465-472.

Dube SR et al. Long-term consequences of childhood sexual abuse by gender of victim. *American Journal of Preventive Medicine 28(5).*

Easton, D. & Liszt, C. (1997) *The Ethical Slut: A Guide to Infinite Sexual Possibilities* Greenery Press CA.

Edwards, E. (1993) Development of a New Scale for Measuring Compulsive Buying Behavior *Financial Counseling and Planning*, 4, 67-85.

Edwards, W. (2009) *Living a Life I Love: Healing from Sexual Compulsivity, Sexual Addiction, Sexual Avoidance and other Sexual Health Concerns*. CreateSpace:Seattle

Edwards, W. (2012) Using a Sexual Health Model to conceptualize cybersex treatment. *Journal of Sexual Compulsivity and Addiction*, manuscript in preparation.

Edwards, W. (2009) Sexual Health and the EA Professional. *Journal of Employee Assistance, 39:2*, 114.

Edwards, W. (2004) *Measuring Sexual Health: Development Of The Sexual Health Inventory*. A Dissertation Submitted To The Faculty Of The Graduate School Of The University Of Minnesota.

Edwards, W. & Coleman E. (2004) Defining sexual health: A descriptive overview. *Archives of Sexual Behavior, 33*(3), 189-195.

Edwards, W., Delmonico, D and Griffin E. (2011) *Cybersex Unplugged: Finding Sexual Health in an Electronic World*. CreateSpace:Seattle

Elliott, D., Mok, D. & Briere, J (2004) Adult Sexual Assault: Prevalence, Symptomatology, and Sex Differences in the General Population, *Journal of Traumatic Stress, 17(3)*, 203-211.

Facing facts: Sexual health for America's adolescents. (1995) D. W. Haffner (Ed.), New York: Sexuality Information and Education Council of the United States (SIECUS).

Feldman, M. & Meyer, I (2007) Eating Disorders in Diverse Lesbian, Gay, and Bisexual Populations *International Journal of Eating Disorders, 40*, 218–226, doi: 10.1002/eat.20360

Ferree, M. (2001) Females and Sex Addiction: Myths and Diagnostic Implications. *Sexual Addiction & Compulsivity, 8(3/4)* 287-300.

Fisher, B., Cullen, F. & Turner M. (2000) The Sexual Victimization of College Women. National Institute of Justice.

Fisher, W. & Barak, A. (2001) Internet pornography: A social psychological perspective on Internet sexuality. *Journal of Sex Research, 38(4)*, 312-323. doi:10.1080/00224490109552102

Illinois Institute for Addiction Recovery (2008) What behaviors indicate compulsive shopping and spending? http://www.addictionrecov.org/spendwhat.htm

Goodman, A. (2001) What's in a Name? Terminology for Designating a Syndrome of Driven Sexual Behavior. *Sexual Addiction & Compulsivity, 8(3/4)*, 191-213.

Gudelunas, D. (2005) Talking taboo: Newspaper advice columns and sexual discourse. *Sexuality & Culture: An Interdisciplinary Quarterly, 9(1)*, 62-87.

Hammack, P. (2005) The Life Course Development of Human Sexual Orientation: An Integrative Paradigm, *Human Development, 48(5)*, 267-290.

Hedgepeth, E. (2000) From Margin to Center: Sexuality Education As a Model for Teaching in a Democracy, *Journal of Sex Education & Therapy, 25(2/3)*, 137-146.

Mallon, S. (2002) Developing a Positive Sexuality Education in the Churches, *British Journal of Theological Education, 12 (2)*, 133-144.

Maltz, W. & Maltz, L (2010) *The Porn Trap: the essential guide to overcoming problems caused by pornography*. Harper Paperback

Meyer, M. (2005) Drawing the sexuality card: Teaching, researching, and living bisexuality. *Sexuality & Culture: An Interdisciplinary Quarterly, 9(1)*, 3-13.

Money, J. (1993) Lovemaps. Prometheus Books, New York. Green, R. Sissy Boys.

Morin, J. *(1996) The Erotic Mind: Unlocking the Inner Sources of Passion and Fulfillment.* Harper Paperbacks

Kaminski, P., Chapman, B., Haynes, S. & Own, L. (2005) Body image, eating behaviors, and attitudes toward exercise among gay and straight men. *Eating Behaviors, 6(3)*, 179-187.

Kalichman, S. (2005) The Other Side of the Healthy Relationships Intervention: Mental Health Outcomes and Correlates of Sexual Risk Behavior Change, *AIDS Education & Prevention; Supplement A, 17*, 66-75.

Kasl, C. (1991) *Women, Sex, and Addiction: A Search for Love and Power*, Harper Perennial

Kelly, M., Strassberg, D. & Turner, C. (2004) Communication and Associated Relationship Issues in Female Anorgasmia. *Journal of Sex & Marital Therapy, 30(4)* 263-276.

Klausner JD, Wolf W, Fischer-Ponce L, Zolt I, Katz MH. (2000) Tracing a syphilis outbreak through cyberspace. *Journal of American Medical Association, 284*, 447-9.

Koch, P., Mansfield, P., Thurau, D. & Carey, M. (2005) Feeling Frumpy": The Relationships Between Body Image and Sexual Response Changes in Midlife Women. *Journal of Sex Research, 42(3)*, 215-223.

Kim, A., McFarland, W., Yu, F. & Klausner, J. (2000) Cybersex.net: Sexual networks over the Internet, Silicon Valley, 1999-2000. Abstracts of the XIII international AIDS conference, Durban, South Africa, 9-14.

Kinsey, A. (1948) *Sexual behavior in the human male*. Philadelphia: W.B. Saunders Company.

Kinsey, A. (1953) *Sexual behavior in the human female*. Philadelphia: W.B. Saunders Company.

Lesieur, H. & Blume, S. (2008) The South Oaks Gambling Screen (SOGS) located at: http://www.addictionrecov.org/southoak.htm

Leiblum, S. (2003) Sex-starved marriages sweeping the US. *Sexual & Relationship Therapy, 18(4),* 427-428,

Mellody, P., Wells-Miller, A., Miller, J. Keith (2003) *Facing Co Dependency*. HarperOne

Mellody, P., Wells-Miller, A., Miller, J. Keith (2003) *Facing Love Addiction*. HarperOne

Melby, T. (2001) Childhood Sexuality. *Contemporary Sexuality, 35(12)* 1-3.

Meston, C. & Buss, D. (2007) Why Humans Have Sex. *Archives of Sexual Behavior* 36, 477–507, doi: 10.1007/s10508-007-9175-2

Meyer, C. & Blissett, J. (2001) Sexual Orientation and Eating Psychopathology: The Role of Masculinity and Femininity, *International Journal of Eating Disorders, 29(3),* 314-318.

National Institute on Alcohol Abuse and Alcoholism. (1995) *Assessing alcohol problems: A guide for clinicians and researchers* (NIH No. 95-3745). Bethesda, MD: National Institute of Health.

Nusbaum M. (2002) Erectile dysfunction: prevalence, etiology, and major risk factors. *The Journal of the American Osteopathic Association, 10(12),* 1-6.

Nusbaum, M., Lenahan, P. & Sadovsky, R (2005) Sexual health in aging men and women: Addressing the physiologic and psychological sexual changes that occur with age. *Geriatrics, 60(9),* 18-23.

Peplau, L., Frederick, D., Yee, C., Maisel, N., Lever, J. & Ghavami, N. (2009) Body Image Satisfaction in Heterosexual, Gay, and Lesbian Adults, *Archives of Sexual Behavior 38,* 713–725, doi: 10.1007/s10508-008-9378-1

Prevalence of Eating Disorders found at: http://www.eatingdisorderscoalition.org/reports/statistics.html

Robinson, B.E., Bockting, W. O. & Harrell, T. (2002) Masturbation and sexual health: An exploratory study of low income African American women. *Journal of Psychology & Human Sexuality, 14*(2/3), 85-102. Co-published simultaneously in Masturbation as a means of achieving sexual health (Eds.). W. O. Bockting & E. Coleman. Binghamton, N.Y.: The Haworth Press, Inc.

Robinson, B., Bockting, W., Rosser, S., Miner, M. & Coleman, E. (2002). The Sexual health model: Application of a sexological approach to HIV prevention. *Health Education Research, 17*(1), 43-57.

Robinson, B., Munns, R., Weber-Main, A., Lowe, M. & Raymond, N (2011) Application of the Sexual Health Model in the Long-Term Treatment of Hypoactive Sexual Desire and Female Orgasmic Disorder. *Archives of Sexual Behavior, 40:2,* 469-478, doi: 10.1007/s10508-010-9673-5

Rosser, B., Dwyer, M, Coleman, E., Miner, M., Metz, M., Robinson, B. & Bockting, W. (1995) Using sexually explicit material in sex education: an eighteen year comparative analysis. *Journal of Sex Education and Therapy, 21,* 117–128.

Rosser, B., Hatfield, L., Miner, M., Ghiselli, M., Lee, B., Welles, S. & the Positive Connections Team. (2010). Effects of a behavioral intervention to reduce serodiscordant unsafe sex among HIV positive Men who have Sex with Men: The Positive Connections randomized controlled trial study. *Journal of Behavioral Medicine, 33(2),* 147-158, doi: 10.1007/s10865-009-9244-1.

Rosen R., Riley A., Wagner G. Osterloh I., Kirkpatrick J. & Mishra A. (1997) The International Index of Erectile Function (IIEF): a multidimensional scale for assessment of erectile dysfunction. *Urology, 49:* 822-830.

Rosser, S., Bockting, W., Ross, M., Miner, M. & Coleman, E. (2008) The Relationship Between Homosexuality, Internalized Homo-Negativity, and Mental Health in Men Who Have Sex with Men. *Journal of Homosexuality, 55:1,* 1-29, doi: 10.1080/00918360802129394.

Rosser, S., Gobby, J. & Carr, P (1999) The Unsafe Sexual Behavior of Persons Living with HIV: An Empirical Approach to Developing Interventions for Persons Living with HIV. *Journal of Sex Education and Therapy, 24(1/2),* 18-28.

Savin-Williams, R. (2005) The New Gay Teen: Shunning Labels. *Gay & Lesbian Review Worldwide, 12(6,)* 16-19.

Scarce, M (2001) *Male on Male Rape: The hidden toll of stigma and shame*. Basic Books

Schneider, J. (2005) *Back From Betrayal*, Third Edition, Chapin

Schwartz, M. F. & Southern, S. (2000) Compulsive cybersex: The new tea room. *Sexual Addiction & Compulsivity,* 7(1-2), 127-144. doi: 10.1080/10720160008400211

Sex Addicts Recovery Resources http://www.sarr.org/coaddicts/default.htm

Sheils, A. & Caruso, J. (2004) A Reliability Induction and Reliability Generalization Study of the Cage Questionnaire. *Educational and Psychological Measurement, 64(2),* 254-270 doi: 10.1177/0013164403261814

Shively M. & DeCecco, J. (1977) Components of Identity, *Journal of Homosexuality 3(1),* 41-48.

Shulman, J. & Home, S. (2003) The Use of Self-Pleasure: Masturbation and Body Image among African American and European American Women. *Psychology of Women Quarterly. 27(3),* 262-269.

Singer, M. (2002) Childhood Sexuality: An Interpersonal-Intrapsychic Integration. *Contemporary Sexuality, 36(11),* 13-.

Smolak, L. & Murnen, S. (2002) Meta-Analytic Examination of the Relationship Between Child Sexual Abuse and Eating Disorders. *International Journal of Eating Disorders. 31(2)*, 136-15

Stern, S. E. & Handel, A. D. (2001). Sexuality and mass media: The historical context of psychology's reaction to sexuality on the Internet, *Journal of Sex Research, 38(4)*, 283-291 doi: 10.1080/00224490109552099

Turner, C., Villarroel, M., Chromy, J., Eggleston, E. & Rogers, S. (2005) Same-Gender Sex Among U.S. Adults. *Public Opinion Quarterly, 69(3)*, 439-462.

Treur, T., Koperdák, M., Rózsa, S. & Füredi, J. (2005) The impact of physical and sexual abuse on body image in eating disorders. *European Eating Disorders Review, 13(2)*, 106-111.

Tripodi, C. (2006) Long Term Treatment of Partners of Sex Addicts: A Multi-Phase Approach. *Sexual Addiction & Compulsivity*, 13, 269-288.

U.S. Department of Health and Human Services (2001) *The surgeon general's call to action to promote sexual health and responsible sexual behavior*. Rockville, MD.

Maltz, W. (2003) Treating the Sexual Intimacy Concerns of Sexual Abuse Survivors. *Contemporary Sexuality, 37(7)*, i-vii.

West, S. & Vinikoor, L, Zolnoun, D. (2004) Systematic Review of the Literature on Female Sexual Dysfunction Prevalence and Predictors. *Annual Review of Sex Research, 15*, 40-172.

Wingood, G., Di Clemente, R., Harrington, K. & Davies, S. (2002) Body Image and African American Females' Sexual Health. *Journal of Women's Health & Gender-Based Medicine, 11(5)* 433-439.

Violence against women (2008) located at: http://www.4woman.gov/violence/types/sexual.cfm

Welcome to the Drug Abuse Screening Test (DAST) (2008) http://counsellingresource.com/quizzes/drug-abuse/index.html.

World Association of Sexology's declaration of sexual rights. (1999) First declared at the 13th World Congress of Sexology, 1997, Valencia, Spain. Revised and approved by the General Assembly of World Association for Sexology on August 26, 1999, during the 14th World Congress of Sexology, Hong Kong, People's Republic of China.

World Health Organization (2002) Gender and reproductive rights, glossary, sexual health. Retrieved on July 11, 2003, from http://www.who.int/reproductive-health/gender/glossary.html.

End Notes

[1] Robinson, B. E., Uhl G., Miner, M., Bockting, W. O., Scheltema, K. E., Rosser, B. R. S., & Westover, B. (2002). Evaluation of a sexual health approach to prevent HIV among low income, urban, primarily African American

[2] If you want to read additional resources, please read *Slowing Down to the Speed of Life* by Carlson and Bailey, *Flow: The Psychology of Optimal Experience* by Csikszentmihalyi, and *Blink: The Power of Thinking Without Thinking* by Gladwell, and The *Power of Now* by Tolle.

[3] See Malcom Gladwell, *Blink*

[4] Bradshaw, John (1998) Healing the Shame that Binds You. HCI

[5] In a few rare circumstances, the external genitalia may be confusing. For more information, search out the term "intersex" on the Internet.

[6] National Institute on Alcohol Abuse and Alcoholism. (1995). *Assessing alcohol problems: A guide for clinicians and researchers* (NIH No. 95-3745). Bethesda, MD: National Institute of Health

[7] Cotton, M. Ball, C., & Robinson, P (2003) Four Simple Questions Can Help Screen for Eating Disorders *Journal General Internal Medicine*, 18(1): *53–56*.doi: 10.1046/j.1525-1497.2003.20374.x.

[8] Adapted from http://www.helpguide.org/mental/suicide_help.htm)

[9] Fisher, Cullen & Turner, 2000

[10] Dube, 2005.

[11] Scarce, 2001.

[12] Adapted from Body Love: Learning to Like Our Looks and Ourselves, Rita Freeman, Ph.D.

[13] Meston, C. & Buss, D. (2007) Why Humans Have Sex. *Archives of Sexual Behavior* 36, 477–507. DOI 10.1007/s10508-007-9175-2